International Handbook
of Arrhythmia

International Handbook
of Arrhythmia

Ronald WF Campbell

Professor of Cardiology, University of Newcastle-upon-Tyne, UK

MARCEL DEKKER, INC.   NEW YORK · BASEL · HONG KONG

ISBN: 0-8247-9819-8

This book is printed on acid-free paper.

Marcel Dekker, Inc.
270 Madison Avenue, New York, New York   10016

Current printing (last digit):
10 9 8 7 6 5 4 3 2 1

PRINTED IN THE UNITED STATES OF AMERICA

Despite improving guidelines and our burgeoning knowledge of disease, clinical medicine remains a challenge. Nowhere is this more evident than in the management of cardiac arrhythmias. These events complicate a wide variety of cardiovascular pathologies but are also found in apparently normal individuals. Theoretically, these events can betoken anything from a better than normal prognosis to one that may be measured in only milliseconds. Worse still, distinguishing subtypes of arrhythmias often seems to owe more to artistic appreciation than to scientific analysis. There seems no end to our woes when we consider that in few other medical situations have drugs been so dramatically revealed to be two-edged, bringing sometimes good but at other times catastrophic harm. Such doom and gloom has concealed remarkable advances in arrhythmia diagnosis and management. We fear arrhythmias, yet over the last two decades arrhythmia morbidity and mortality have fallen. While it would be pleasant if credit could be given to electrophysiological advances, in reality the greatest antiarrhythmic impact has come from interventions that preserve and minimize damage to cardiac tissue: thrombolysis, beta-blockers, aspirin, lipid-lowering therapy, ACE inhibitors, and others.

Many cardiac arrhythmias are not associated with degenerative cardiac diseases, or indeed with any other cardiac pathology. Their basis lies in remnants of cardiac tissue that have persisted abnormally since birth. Over 90% of all regular narrow QRS tachycardias ("supra" ventricular tachycardias) fall within this category. Appreciation of their anatomy has spawned the dramatic advance of radiofrequency (RF) ablation. Another nonpharmacological therapeutic advance is the implantable cardioverter defibrillator (ICD), which, to those of use who used the external defibrillators of 20 years ago, seems to defy all that we learned about energy requirements for defibrillation. There is no doubt that this device can save life, but it is not a therapy to be dispensed lightly.

Arrhythmia management is not just about spectacular pharmacoelectrophysiology, precision lesion placement, or microelectronics. These interventions must be prescribed and deployed by physicians who understand arrhythmias, who can accurately diagnose arrhythmias, who can infer the susceptibility of the arrhythmia, and who can accurately access the implication of the arrhythmia. This small handbook could never impart all that information, but if offers the key points: terminology, anatomy, mechanism, ECG appearance, and management. If you use any one or all of these features, I hope that this is one book that is always in your hand.

Ronald W. F. Campbell

Contents

CHAPTER 1

Introduction

Cardiac arrhythmias are a common accompaniment of a variety of cardiac diseases. Even in health, it is normal to find that stable sinus rhythm is not a universal finding. Variations of RR interval are common, as are occasional atrial and ventricular ectopic beats (1).

Cardiac arrhythmias become important when they cause symptoms, threaten life, or are indicative of an adverse prognosis. In the last 20 years, most attention has been paid to ventricular ectopic beats. They have prognostic implications for a variety of cardiac pathologies, but it has become clear that their suppression is not necessarily rewarded with an improved outlook for affected patients (2).

In the clinical management of arrhythmias, an accurate diagnosis is essential. The impact of the arrhythmia on symptoms and/or prognosis must be established. Only after determining these two features can the need and the aim of intervention be decided. When treatment is pharmacological, the range of likely effective drugs should be reviewed and the one, or ones, with the best risk–benefit ratio should be chosen as the first-line therapy.

Dramatic advances in nonpharmacological therapies dictate that physicians managing arrhythmias know when to abandon drug approaches in favor of radiofrequency (RF) ablation, map-directed antiarrhythmic surgery, or the implantable cardioverter-defibrillator.

CHAPTER 2

Sinus Rhythm

The sinus node lies in the superior part of the right atrium at its junction with the superior vena cava. It is a complex and little-understood structure. It is the heart's dominant pacemaker. Its intrinsic rate is modulated by a variety of neurohormonal influences to cause rate acceleration in situations of increased demand for cardiac output, e.g., on exercise, during pregnancy, and with emotion. Rate increases are caused by a combination of increased sympathetic tone (with a balanced withdrawal of vagal tone) and the effects of circulating catecholamines. An increased rate of sinus node discharge also occurs in pathological situations such as hyperthyroidism, fever, and anemia. In these conditions, the behavior of the sinus node is not abnormal; it is responding appropriately to external driving influences.

Slowing of the sinus node occurs with withdrawal of sympathetic activity and an increase in vagal or parasympathetic tone. This occurs naturally with sleep, and in normal individuals there is an impressive diurnal variation of sinus rate, with the lowest rates being recorded at night (Figure 1). Rapid eye movement (REM) sleep, however, is associated with sympathetic activation and at these times an increase in sinus node discharge rate is seen.

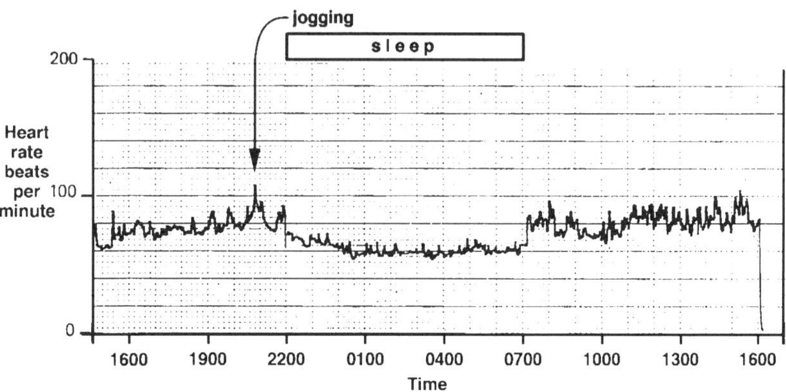

Figure 1:   Heart rate plot of a healthy subject. Note the differences between daytime and nightime rates and the reduced rate fluctuations at night.

NORMAL SINUS RHYTHM

Classically, normal sinus rhythm is arbitrarily defined as a rate between 60 and 100 beats per minute. Lower rates are termed sinus bradycardia and faster rates sinus tachycardia. These definitions are acceptable only if sinus node rate variations outside this band range are not automatically considered pathological. In healthy young adults, nocturnal sinus rates may fall to 40 beats per minute or even lower and be quite normal. Similarly, low daytime resting sinus node rates are found in young, well-trained individuals and in athletes in particular. Sinus tachycardia occurs at some point in most 24-hour ECG recordings of normal individuals except perhaps in those leading a very sedentary existence. A moment's consideration of the heart rate targets used in Bruce exercise stress testing shows that quite rapid sinus rates are expected, and are achieved by normal subjects and cardiac patients alike (3).

The major reason for sinus rate variation is as a control mechanism for cardiac output. In the athletically trained, remarkable increases in cardiac output can be achieved by changes in stroke volume with little change in heart rate. In most normal individuals, however, heart rate acceleration is the dominant method for increasing cardiac output. At very high rates, the time available for ventricular filling becomes so abbreviated that cardiac output may fall. There is thus an "upper rate limit" beyond which little or no hemodynamic benefit occurs. The mechanism of this rate limit is not understood in humans, but in response to physiological stimuli, the maximum achievable heart rate seems to approximate to the ideal "upper rate."

SINUS ARRHYTHMIA AND THE PR INTERVAL

Deriving the hemodynamic benefit of an increased heart rate demands more than mere acceleration of rate. Atrial and ventricular contraction time must be optimized for rate. This is achieved by modulation of atrioventricular (AV) node behavior. With higher heart rates, AV conduction time is abbreviated. Invasive electrophysiological studies show this effect to occur within the AV node, as reflected by AH (atrial to His bundle activation time) changes with the HV interval (His bundle to ventricular myocardial activation time) being almost unchanged by rate. This AV nodal effect is seen on the surface ECG as a PR change. A normal PR interval is usually defined as between 120 and 200 ms (0.12 to 0.20 s or between three and five small ECG paper squares at a paper speed of 25 squares per ms). PR intervals longer than 200 ms (or 220 ms, as suggested by some authorities) are conventionally described as first-degree AV block. A more sophisticated definition of first-degree AV block would consider the sinus rate at which the PR interval was measured. This has particular relevance in healthy young individuals, who may have low resting heart rates and in whom a PR interval of 260 ms or more may be normal.

SINUS TACHYCARDIA

An appropriate sinus tachycardia is present when the sinus discharge rate is more rapid than is demanded by the cardiac output needs. Many situations reflect extracardiac pathology, for example, hyperthyroidism, anemia, or a catecholamine-secreting tumor. Very rarely, a pathological sinus tachycardia may be generated by an abnormality in the sinus node. The findings are of an abnormally fast sinus rate. The P waves are normal, as the origin of the impulse is the sinus node and spread of atrial activation is normal. Unlike normal sinus tachycardia, pathological sinus tachycardia does not show modulations with time. A 24-hour ECG, for instance, would show markedly reduced nocturnal slowing, or none at all. Such a finding, however, is not unique to pathological intrinsic sinus tachycardia; similar features may be seen in hyperthyroidism and some situations of abnormal catecholamine secretion. Intrinsic pathological sinus tachycardia is very uncommon. If suspected, sophisticated investigation by invasive programmed electrical stimulation may be needed to differentiate it from atrial tachycardia and secondary sinus tachycardia.

Atrial Fibrillation

Atrial fibrillation (AF), an important and common cardiac arrhythmia, is associated with a variety of cardiac and noncardiac diseases. Its prevalence increases with age (4)—community studies suggest that AF is present in up to 1% of an apparently normal population over the age of 70 years. Such a finding might encourage clinical complacency over diagnosis and management of this arrhythmia, but AF is associated with hemodynamic detriment and, more importantly, with a significant risk of thromboembolism (5).

MECHANISM AND RATE CONSEQUENCE

AF is probably the consequence of multiple macro reentrant circuits within the atria (Figure 2). Some evidence suggests that the left atrium may be more important than the right in this regard, but this is far from proven. The atrial rhythm is described as "chaotic" and the surface ECG P waves are lost, to be replaced with an undulating irregular baseline (Figure 3). In reality, the rhythm is probably not truly chaotic—in neither a mathematical nor a clinical sense. The fast irregular atrial rhythm bombards the AV node, which is incapable of transmitting all the impulses to the His-Purkinje network and the ventricular myocardium. This is fortunate because the atrial "rate" may exceed 400 beats per minute. Nonetheless, the ventricular response rates achieved are usually much too fast for hemodynamic efficacy.

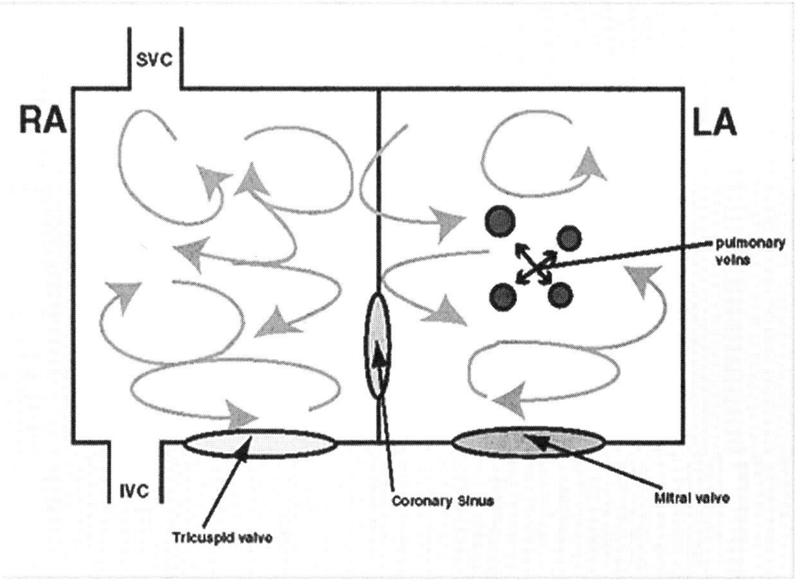

Figure 2: Diagram of the interlacing wavelets of reentry responsible for atrial fibrillation.

Cardiac output is compromised, not just by the rate alone but also by the loss of atrial transport (there is no coordinated effective atrial contraction during AF) and by the irregularity of the ventricular response. From these considerations it is clear that while management by ventricular rate control will offer some advantage to the affected patient, only restoration of sinus rhythm will address all of the hemodynamically detrimental effect of AF.

THROMBOEMBOLISM

Thromboembolism is a major risk of AF. There is stasis of blood in the fibrillating atria, particularly in the auricular appendings. Without anticoagulation there is a risk of systemic embolization from the left atrium. Theoretically, there is also a risk of pulmonary embolism from the right atrium

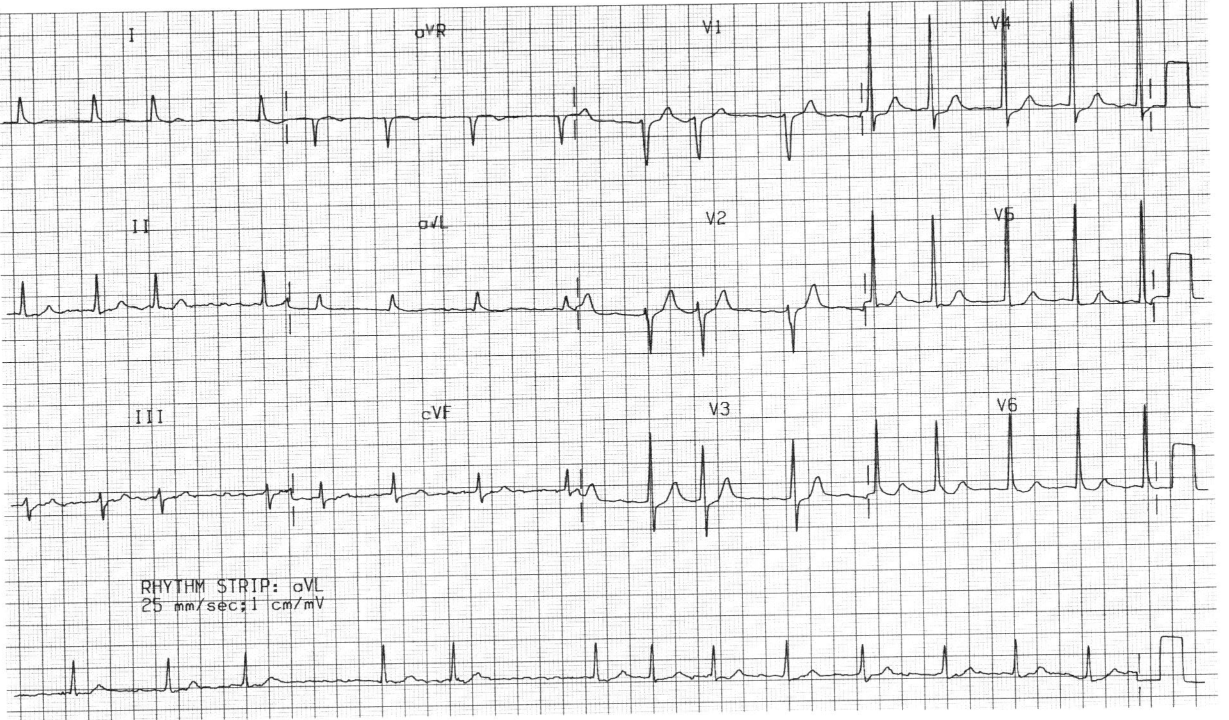

Figure 3: 12-lead ECG of AF. Note the absence of P waves and the irregular narrow QRS complexes. The average ventricular rate is 100 beats per minute. The patient is on digoxin; this probably explains the nonspecific ST- and T-wave changes in V3–6.

but, for whatever reason, this is less commonly diagnosed clinically. The risk of thromboembolism is not just dependent on the rhythm; the associated cardiac disease has a major modulating influence. For instance, the thromboembolic risk of lone AF (AF without evidence of structural heart disease) is only modestly greater than for similar individuals in sinus rhythm. In contrast, the risk of thromboembolism is very high in those whose AF is associated with rheumatic mitral valve disease.

The prophylactic approach to thromboembolism is not simple; the risks and benefits of therapy need careful and individual appraisal. Warfarin has been proven effective in preventing thromboembolism. Aspirin, however, offers relatively weak protection and is indicated only when warfarin is contraindicated or in very special circumstances of low risk—for instance, in "lone" AF, in which there is truly no structural heart disease.

CATEGORIES OF ATRIAL FIBRILLATION

On the surface ECG, all AF looks similar. There are no P waves; the baseline is irregular and shows rapid, low-voltage deflection; and there is a fast, irregular ventricular response. In fact, there may be ECG subtypes of AF with clinical relevance but currently, little effort is made to distinguish these. Examples might be the coarse and fine fibrillatory wave patterns that attracted cardiological attention some 40 or 50 years ago. These may correlate with the numbers and size of the intra-atrial reentrant circuits but this has yet to be established.

Many attempts have been made to classify AF. The variables considered include associated disease and the onset and attack pattern. Thus, the following types might be distinguished: lone (no structural disease), ischemic, rheumatic, and cardiomyopathic; vagal, sympathetic, paroxysmal, persistent, and permanent. Each scheme has merits. Not surprisingly, much is to be gained by combining these sets to more accurately define AF subtypes. This exercise is not merely intellectual; there is increasing evidence that various subtypes have differing therapeutic needs.

ASSOCIATED DISEASE

Disease processes that encourage AF are those that increase atrial wall tension, including mitral valve disease (of any etiology), hypertension, left ventricular hypertrophy, aortic valve disease (late), and any cause of heart failure. Ischemic heart disease may also cause AF. The mechanism may be either through atrial stretch or by direct ischemic and/or infarct damage to the atrial myocardium. Hyperthyroidism also causes AF. This is a direct consequence of the atrial electrophysiological effects of the abnormally elevated thyroid hormones.

Establishing the nature and severity of the etiological disease is important because restoration and maintenance of sinus rhythm are unlikely unless the underlying pathology is ameliorated. Thus, relief of valve obstruction or reduced regurgitation, lowering of blood pressure, management of ischemia, and aggressive therapy for heart failure can all play a useful supportive antiarrhythmic role.

In addition, the greater the structural abnormality of the atria, the more chance there is for blood stasis and clot formation. Managing the underlying disease has consequences for reducing the risks of thromboembolism.

AUTONOMIC ASSOCIATIONS

An attractive concept for distinguishing types of paroxysmal AF came with the suggestion that sympathetically and parasympathetically modulated types could be identified by the history of the event or, better, by detailed analysis of a 24-hour ECG recording encompassing the onset of a paroxysm (6). Sympathetically modulated AF would occur in the setting of increased sympathetic tone, for example, during exercise or emotion. Pre-event shortening of R-R intervals would be seen, either overtly or subtly, on Holter monitor recordings. Beta-blockers would be expected to be useful therapy, and indeed, when such sympathetically modulated paroxysms occur consistently, these drugs are useful. Parasympathetically modulated AF should occur at rest, at night, or following exercise. This form is unusual. No specific antiarrhythmic interventions have proved useful, although some anecdotes support a role for disopyramide, which has antiadrenergic actions. In other situations, where cardiac slowing is more apparent, there may be a role for antibradycardia pacing.

Attractive as the concept of automatically modulated AF is, reality has shown that clear distinction of these categories is difficult and that consistent patterns in individual patients are uncommon. Nocturnal paroxysms, for instance, may reflect vagal tone or, with REM sleep, sympathetic activation. Similarly, the relationship with exercise is rarely secure.

ATTACK PATTERN

There are numerous schemes for classifying AF by the pattern of attacks. Categorization into paroxysmal, persistent, and permanent AF is simple and clinically useful (Figure 4). *Paroxysmal* AF, by definition, will stop spontaneously, although perhaps a time definition is needed for this type. In practice it may be unnecessary; most true paroxysms do not last longer than 24 hours. An attack lasting longer should be labeled *persistent*. This means that the patient, when seen, is still in AF. Restoration of sinus rhythm is desirable and may be possible. In contrast, *permanent* AF will not correct to sinus rhythm; ventricular rate control is the appropriate strategy.

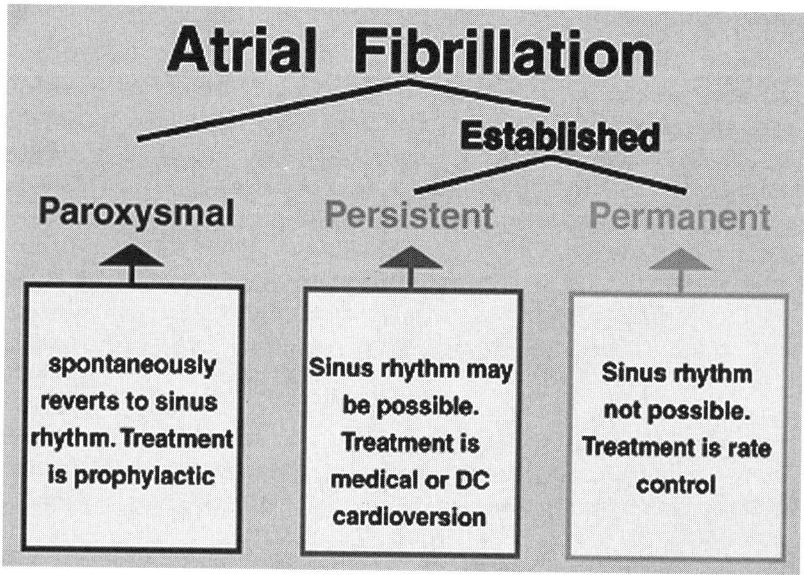

Figure 4: Subtypes of atrial fibrillation.

MANAGEMENT PRINCIPLES

The management of AF has been unnecessarily complicated. Almost every antiarrhythmic drug can influence either the arrhythmia itself or the AV nodal conduction of the fibrillatory impulses. Regrettably, there is no consensus on the drugs that have a first-line indication. Rather than try to establish a strategy that is rigid and will inevitably find dissenters, it is possible to recommend a group of therapies with special efficacy for specific aspects and types of AF. These agents reduce the number of circulating wavelets of reentry from the minimum of six or seven needed to sustain the arrhythmia (7). They either prolong the wavelength of the circuit (sotalol, amiodarone) or block the circuit (propafenone, flecainide) (Figure 5).

The aim of management of any type of AF is to establish a "satisfactory clinical situation with or without anticoagulation or aspirin depending upon the perceived thromboembolic risk." This rather vague therapeutic aim can be criticized, yet most practicing clinicians can recognize this "endpoint" and would acknowledge the therapeutic freedom it provides.

PAROXYSMAL ATRIAL FIBRILLATION

For those patients with paroxysmal AF whose attacks are infrequent, short-lived, and well tolerated, no therapy other than reassurance may be necessary. When symptoms become a problem, therapy should be directed at reducing or abolishing the paroxysm. The value of shortening the duration of paroxysms, or of lengthening the time between paroxysms, should not be underestimated. Achieving these endpoints may require quite modest doses of drugs that in full dose might not be well tolerated. The antiarrhythmic drugs with best efficacy and acceptable safety for paroxysms are the class 1c drugs propafenone and flecainide, the beta-blockers, and amiodarone. Although many other drugs have some efficacy for this indication, in clinical studies they have proved to be less successful.

In very extreme situations in which paroxysmal AF will not respond to drug therapy and when symptoms are severe, a nonpharmacological approach may be necessary. Radiofrequency (RF) ablation of the AV node is the best investigated option (8). It is not a procedure to be lightly undertaken because the patient will require permanent pacing, preferably with a sophisticated mode-switching dual-chamber generator. This therapy, while

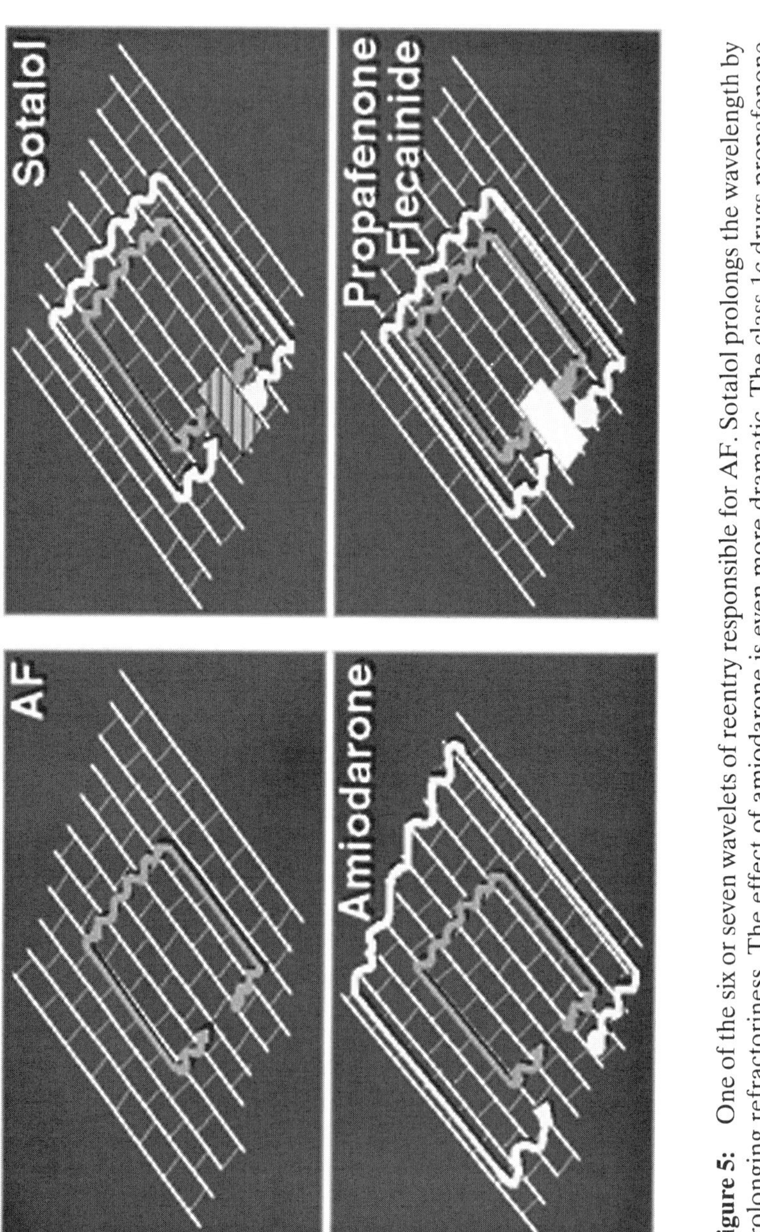

Figure 5: One of the six or seven wavelets of reentry responsible for AF. Sotalol prolongs the wavelength by prolonging refractoriness. The effect of amiodarone is even more dramatic. The class 1c drugs propafenone and flecainide block the reentry circuit primarily at its slow anisotropic phase as the wavelet crosses the line of atrial cells. Propafenone may also modestly prolong refractoriness. Either mechanism—prolonging refractoriness or blocking the circuit—reduces the number of wavelets to below the critical six or seven required to maintain AF.

effective for selected patients, is palliative. Patients will still have prolonged AF, and some may be aware of the change in atrial rhythm despite the fact that the pacemaker will convert from DDD pacing to VVI(R). In addition, patients will remain at risk of thromboembolism, requiring consideration of appropriate prophylaxis.

PERSISTENT ATRIAL FIBRILLATION

In patients with persistent AF, restoration of sinus rhythm *may* be possible. Clearly, if sinus rhythm can be re-established this is the best option for the patient. Therapy then is cardioversion, either electrical or pharmacological, with or without subsequent prophylaxis against recurrences.

It is in this group of patients that the greatest problems arise with respect to reducing the risk of thromboembolism. If AF has been present less than 24 hours, most would agree that either medical or electrical cardioversion can proceed without anticoagulation. Others might demand that an echo (preferably a transesophageal echo) should show no evidence of intra-atrial clot, but in practice this technique may not be readily available. Moreover, it is relatively invasive, and there is no guarantee of cardioversion safety even if no clot is revealed. Prior to DC conversion, any arrhythmogenic factors that can be modified should be. For example, electrolytes and acid-base balance should be corrected; heart failure and ischemia should be managed. Under a light general anesthetic with full resuscitation facilities (synchronized defibrillator, temporary pacing facility) at hand, and with continuous ECG monitoring, an anteroposterior discharge of 100 Joules should be given. If unsuccessful, 200 Joules and, if necessary, the full output of the defibrillator should be tried. Shocks *must* be synchronized to the R wave of the ECG. There are different recommendations for energy delivery; this one implies a maximum of three shocks at escalating energy. Although, theoretically, delivering a shock of the same energy after an unsuccessful one may prove successful, there is probably little detriment to the use of a bigger shock. This scheme has the attraction of minimizing the procedural time and reducing the number of potentially thrombogenic shocks.

Pharmacological cardioversion may be achieved by a variety of drugs. Quinidine has been used in the past, but toxic reactions were not uncommon (9). Propafenone (10), flecainide (11), and amiodarone (12) are effective for restoring sinus rhythm and can do so with an acceptably low incidence of unwanted effects. Given parenterally, they can offer a relatively rapid effect and, if used in this way within the 24-hour window of AF onset, anticoagulation may not be necessary. When AF has continued beyond 24 hours or when drug cardioversion is not quickly achieved, anticoagulation is necessary and should be given for 4 weeks before DC cardioversion and continued for at least 8 weeks after successful restoration of sinus rhythm.

After restoring sinus rhythm, a decision must be made as to whether drug prophylaxis of further events is appropriate. There is a good case for giving no therapy after the first attack since in up to 50% of patients there are no recurrences. If another event does occur, then there is a clear mandate to use drug prophylaxis. Therapies to be considered include propafenone, flecainide, amiodarone, and the beta-blockers.

PERMANENT ATRIAL FIBRILLATION

Sinus rhythm cannot be restored in patients with permanent AF. Some patients may first have been categorized as having persistent AF but attempts at restoring sinus rhythm failed. The management strategy for these patients is ventricular rate control. For many years, digoxin has been the drug of choice for this purpose. Digoxin increases refractoriness of the AV node, reducing the number of impulses transmitted from the fibrillating atria to the ventricles. It is an effective therapy for controlling the resting rate response, but on exercise rate control may not be ideal. Very little is known about optimal rate control of AF, but in some patients, particularly those with impaired effort capacity who show "excessive" rate responses, the addition of either a beta-blocker (13) or a calcium antagonist (14) (diltiazem or verapamil) may be useful.

When drug control of the ventricular response rate is ineffective, RF ablation of the AV node should be considered. The technique is straightforward, but it leaves the patient pacemaker-dependent. A VVIR system is the appropriate generator for implantation. There are early reports that RF modification of the AV node may be possible such that the rate response is controlled and AV conduction is not interrupted (15). For the moment, this management strategy should be considered experimental. Both RF procedures leave the atria fibrillating, as does drug therapy for rate control.

For all patients, anticoagulation or aspirin should be considered as prophylaxis against thromboembolism.

SURGERY

Dissatisfaction with drug management of recalcitrant forms of AF has prompted development of surgical procedures that may help selected patients. In the best-developed technique, the Maze procedure, the atria are surgically divided into strips that are too small to contain a complete reentrant circuit (16). When the strips are sewn together, the suture lines offer lines of conduction block that constrain the electrical impulses to a carefully designated route from the sinus node to the AV node. It is a considerable surgical procedure. Moderate success rates have been reported, but there has been a relatively high incidence of sinus-node dysfunction necessitating pacemaker implantation. There is great interest in simplifying the surgical technique and in trying to reproduce the procedure using catheter-delivered RF energy. At present, these are evolving procedures that may yet mature to become a more general part of AF management.

CHAPTER 4

Atrial Flutter

Atrial flutter is usually produced by a single macro-reentrant loop of electrical activity in the right atrium (Figure 6) (17). As such, it is fundamentally different from atrial fibrillation, yet until recently, AF and atrial flutter were often considered the same entities.

Atrial flutter is relatively rare. Many patients with AF have short periods when their ECG shows more coordinated atrial activity, but this is probably merely a chance coalescence of the six or seven wavelets of reentry that then briefly mimic the single wave responsible for atrial flutter. Additionally, as atrial fibrillation terminates, it may do so by a progressive reduction in numbers of wavelets, passing through a phase of a mere one or two wavelets prior to termination. Such examples have earned the designation *flutter-fibrillation*, but this is not a clinically separate entity.

ANATOMY

The reentrant loop responsible for atrial flutter has an important zone of slow conduction situated near the orifice of the coronary sinus. Electrical activity may circulate in either direction around the loop. When it travels craniocaudally from the sinus-node region to the AV node on the anterior wall of the RA, returning posteriorly, it produces the so-called "common" form of atrial flutter. Circulation in the opposite direction is probably

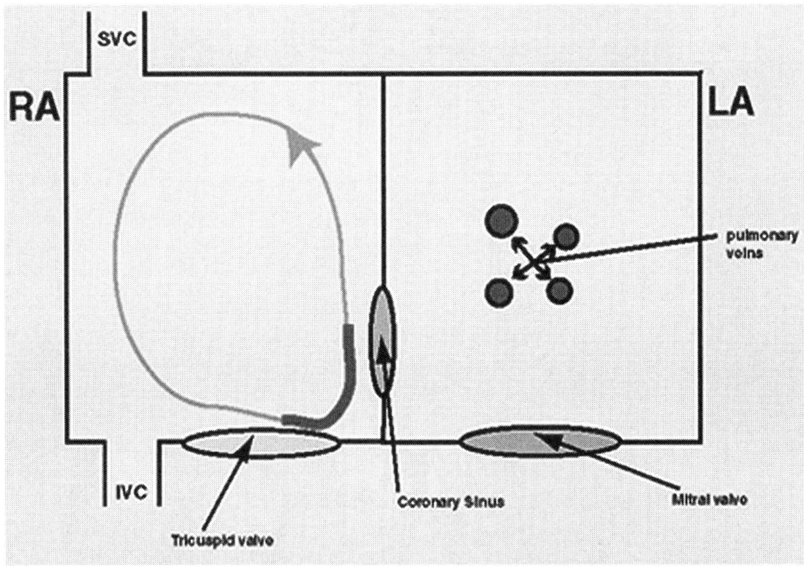

Figure 6:   Diagram of the single right atrial macro-reentrant circuit responsible for atrial flutter.

responsible for the "uncommon" form, although some have suggested that this is a distinct and different entity.

Atrial flutter is associated with structural heart disease, including rheumatic and ischemic heart disease.

DRUG THERAPY

The large macro-reentrant loop with an area of slow conduction poses a major challenge for drug control, and it is no surprise that drug efficacy is low. Slowing conduction in the loop is not enough; conduction block is the goal. This is most likely to occur at the site of abnormally slow conduction and may be achieved with propafenone or flecainide. Prolonging refractori-

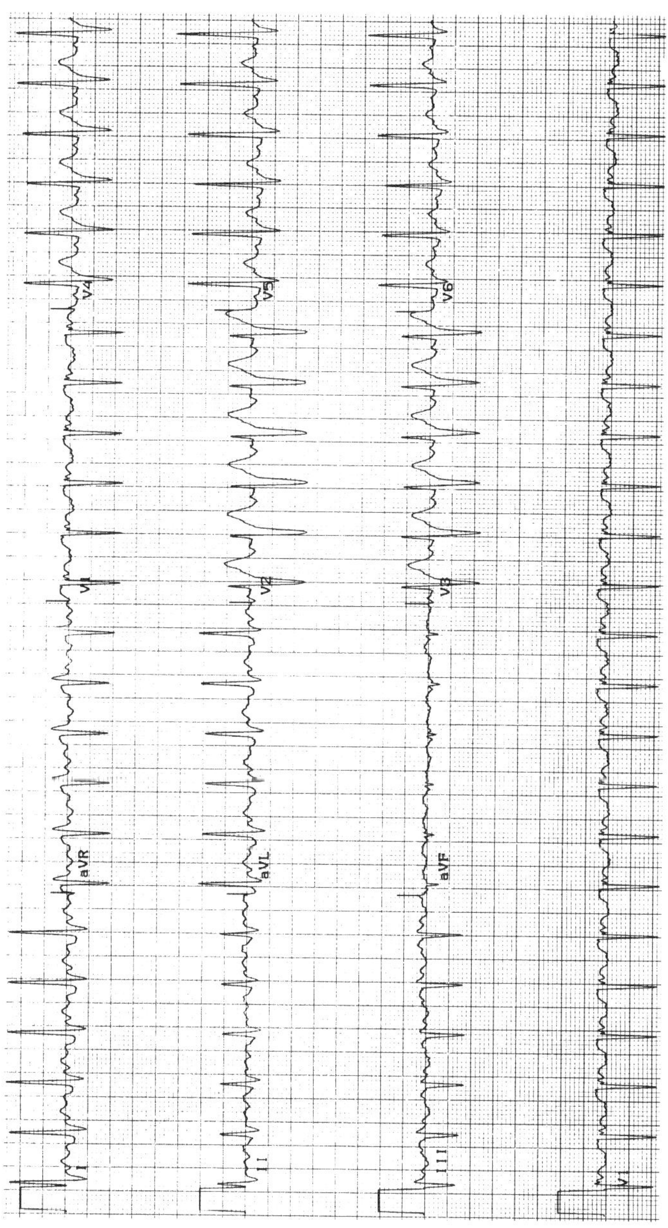

Figure 7: 12-lead ECG of atrial flutter. The flutter rate is 300 beats per minute. There is 2:1 AV conduction, producing a ventricular rate of 150 beats per minute.

ness, as with amiodarone, may be modestly successful. None of these interventions is particularly effective in the acute termination of the arrhythmia, but if programmed catheter stimulation is added, 80 to 90% of events can be stopped.

In atrial flutter, the atrial cycle length is typically 200 to 250 ms (rate 240 to 300 beats per minute) (Figure 7). There is usually 2:1, or even 3:1, conduction at the AV node, with a resulting ventricular rate of 80 to 130 beats per minute. With drug therapy, the atrial cycle may be sufficiently slowed for 1:1 AV conduction to become possible with a sudden increase in the ventricular response rate. This may cause hemodynamic collapse. Digoxin given before administration of other therapy should guard against this possibility, and this approach is now widely practiced.

RADIOFREQUENCY ABLATION

Knowledge of the anatomy of the flutter circuit has led to the development of RF catheter ablation to create complete conduction block in the area of abnormal conduction. A series of RF lesions link the orifice of the coronary sinus, the tricuspid annulus, and the inferior vena cava. Success rates of 80% are reported for restoring stable sinus rhythm (18).

THROMBOEMBOLISM

The risk of thromboembolism in atrial flutter has not been established. Unlike AF, there is some coordinate contraction of the atria, but it is modest and there is considerable scope for stasis. In the presence of structural heart disease, prophylaxis against thromboembolism is advised.

Accessory Pathway Arrhythmias

Muscular accessory atrioventricular connections that offer an alternative to the AV node as a conduction route for impulses between the atria and ventricles were the target of the earliest clinical electrophysiological research. These pathways offered a model of a macro-reentrant tachycardia and permitted the investigation of modes of tachycardia initiation, the effects of antiarrhythmic therapy, and, importantly, the anatomy of the arrhythmia. In some ways, accessory pathway arrhythmias have attracted more attention than they may deserve, yet they are responsible for up to 50% of all sustained narrow QRS tachycardias and for a small but preventable number of arrhythmic deaths. In more recent times, knowledge of these pathways has been largely responsible for the development of curative radiofrequency ablation techniques that are now applied to the management of a great variety of arrhythmias.

ANATOMY

In the normal heart, the only electrical connection between the atria and ventricles is the AV node and His bundle, which penetrates the nonconducting fibrous AV plate of the mitral and tricuspid valve ring. In the process of cardiac development, stray muscular connections may remain and some may be the basis of an electrical connection. Of the pathways that do conduct, some are capable of bidirectional conduction and others of only unidirectional conduction, whether atrioventricular or ventriculoatrial. Accessory atrioventricular muscle connections may occur anywhere on the AV rings. Most are an isolated congenital abnormality, although there is an association of left-sided accessory pathways with mitral valve prolapse and of right-sided pathways with Ebstein's anomaly. Multiple accessory pathways are not rare.

PREVALENCE AND ELECTROCARDIOGRAM EXPRESSION

The prevalence of accessory pathways in the population is not known accurately, but on the basis of surface ECGs, which detect only pathways actively involved in atrioventricular conduction, an incidence of 1 in 1000 apparently normal individuals has been suggested. Accessory pathways may be overt, as when their presence is indicated on the surface ECG by a slurred QRS complex (the delta wave or initial slow component of the QRS is caused by the slow cell-to-cell conduction in myocardium activated by the accessory pathway) and an apparently abbreviated PR interval (Figure 8). Concealed accessory pathways are those either incapable of atrioventricular conduction or that are latent; i.e., atrioventricular conduction is exclusively over the AV node despite the conduction availability of the accessory pathway. This latter situation is seen most often with left lateral accessory pathways that are activated very late in the course of atrial depolarization. The putative location of accessory pathways can be established for the surface ECG when there is maximal pre-excitation (Figure 9).

ARRHYTHMIAS

All types of accessory pathways can support reciprocating tachycardia (sometimes called atrioventricular or AV reentry tachycardia). In this arrhythmia, there is a macro-reentrant loop of cardiac excitation. In the most typical form, *orthodromic reciprocating tachycardia*, activation passes from the atrium through the AV node to the ventricle and returns to the atrium retrogradely over the accessory pathway. The resultant ECG shows a rapid (usually 180 to 220 beats per minute) narrow QRS tachycardia that

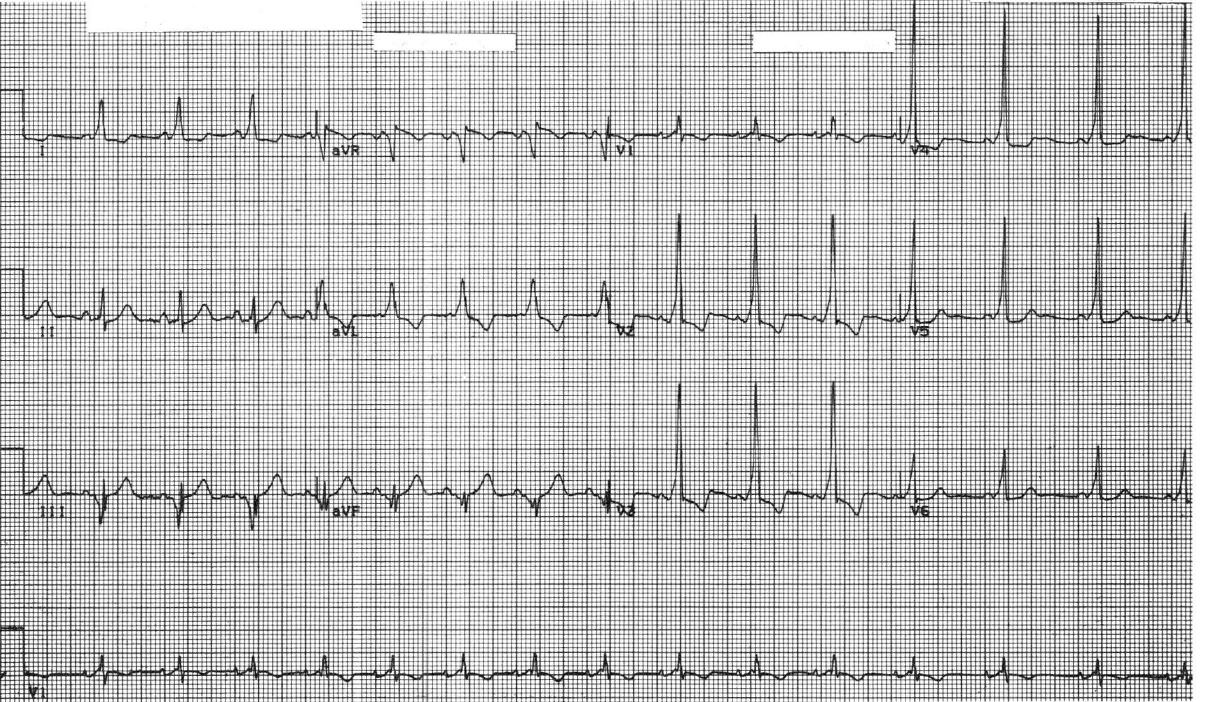

Figure 8: 12-lead ECG of pre-excitation. The onset of the QRS is slurred (the delta wave), especially in leads I, AVL, and V2–6. The QRS in V1 is predominantly positive. The PR interval is short. The pattern of the delta wave is consistent with a left posterior accessory pathway.

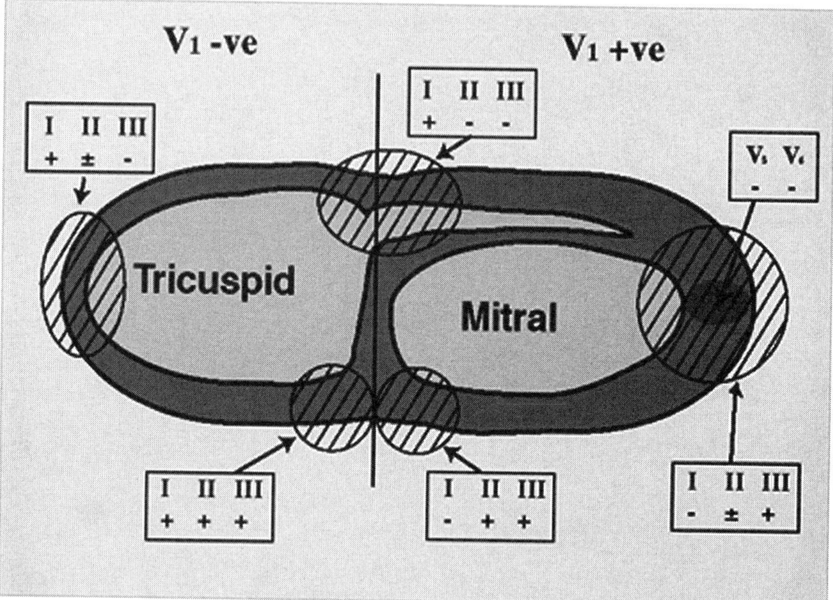

Figure 9: Diagram of the delta-wave polarities associated with specific locations of accessory pathways.

is regular. P waves are usually evident and fall just after the QRS complex such that the PR interval exceeds the RP interval (Figure 10). In the much rarer *antedromic reciprocating tachycardia*, activation is in the opposite direction. The ECG shows a broad slurred QRS complex as ventricular activation is by slow cell-to-cell conduction. The His-Purkinje system plays little or no part in ventricular activation. Since the P waves may be difficult to identify, the ECG is easily mistaken for that of ventricular tachycardia. Prior knowledge of an accessory pathway with a delta wave in sinus rhythm should be a strong clue that the arrhythmia is not ventricular tachycardia.

ACUTE TREATMENT

Both forms of reciprocating tachycardia (orthodromic and antedromic) involve atrial tissue, ventricular tissue, AV nodal tissue, and the accessory

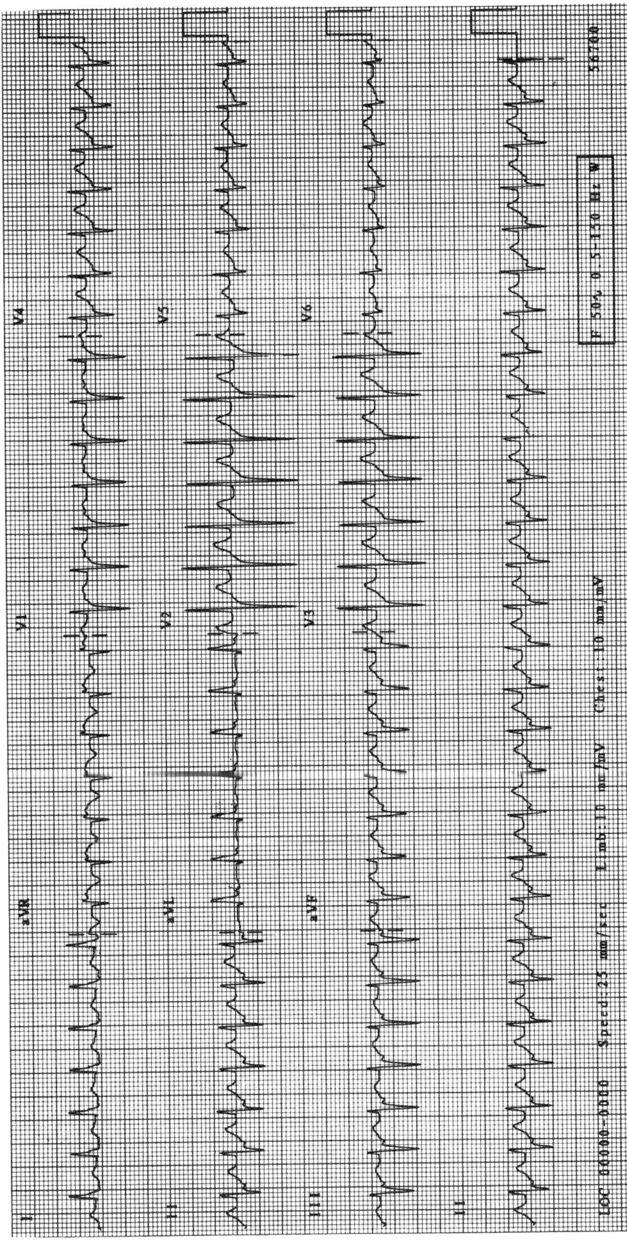

Figure 10: 12-lead ECG of orthodromic reciprocating tachycardia. The rate is 170 beats per minute. Retrograde P waves are seen just after the QRS complexes.

pathway. These rhythms are usually very stable, but the involvement of the AV node within the circuit provides a method of stopping the arrhythmia through increased vagal tone. The Valsalva maneuver or other vagotonic maneuvers such as immersing the face in cold water, drinking cold water, or carotid sinus massage may increase conduction time within the AV node enough to destabilize the circuit and restore sinus rhythm. When these measures fail, pharmacological intervention is appropriate. In the past, verapamil given intravenously has been the drug of choice. It is safe and effective for this indication, but, for reasons of simplicity in the emergency management of a variety of tachycardias, it has been superseded by adenosine (19).

CHRONIC THERAPY

Acute termination of attacks by vagal or pharmacological maneuvers is usually possible, and for some patients with relatively infrequent attacks that are relatively well tolerated, occasional intermittent therapy may be an acceptable management strategy. In most symptomatic patients, prophylaxis is necessary. Although in acute termination the AV node is targeted, for chronic prophylaxis the target should be the accessory pathway. Many antiarrhythmic drugs have utility in patients with reciprocating tachycardia. Since most affected patients are young and would require prolonged therapy, it is important to select the safest effective therapy. Many accessory pathways are sensitive to the class 1c drugs propafenone and flecainide, which can often produce complete block of the pathway. These drugs are good and safe for this indication. In contrast, although quinidine and procainamide have utility, their unwanted effects are sufficiently frequent to preclude their good use. Amiodarone is also effective for the prophylaxis of reciprocating tachycardias. Its not inconsiderable noncardiac toxic effects must be weighed against the benefits of rhythm control. If amiodarone is to be used, the lowest effective dose should be sought.

NONPHARMACOLOGICAL THERAPY

A proportion of reciprocating tachycardias cannot be prevented by drug therapy. In the 1970s, when it had been shown that accessory pathways could be identified by cardiac mapping, a surgical approach was developed. Surgery was recommended for patients whose pathways caused unmanageable symptoms or threatened life and who were unresponsive to or could not tolerate drug therapy. Remarkable success rates are possible, although good results demand a well-trained surgical and electrophysiological team. The surgical procedure is considerable, and a surgical mortality of up to 1% has occurred in some series. Nowadays, almost no surgical division of accessory pathways is undertaken. The technique has been almost completely supplanted by radiofrequency ablation. The position of the accessory pathway is located by intracardiac mapping using a variety of electrode catheters. A specially designed large-tip ablating catheter is then positioned at the accessory pathway and its tip gently heated by the delivery of radiofrequency energy. Success rates exceed 95% and in many series are 99% (20). Fatalities have occurred, but the mortal risk is probably less than 1 in 1000. Not surprisingly, curative radiofrequency ablation is gradually displacing drug management of reciprocating tachycardias.

ATRIAL FIBRILLATION AND ACCESSORY PATHWAY CONDUCTION

In patients with accessory pathways that are capable of atrioventricular conduction, there is a risk that during atrial fibrillation the normal great limiting function of the AV node will be bypassed by conduction over the accessory pathway. Depending on the refractory period of the accessory pathway, rapid and potentially dangerous ventricular response rates may be produced (Figure 11) (21). It might be argued that atrial fibrillation is an uncommon arrhythmia in young individuals who have accessory pathways, but there is good evidence that the pathway itself predisposes to the development of atrial fibrillation.

The acute management of atrial fibrillation with conduction over an accessory pathway to the ventricles resulting in very rapid ventricular response rates does *not* entail the use of drugs that slow AV nodal conduction or increase its refractoriness. Such drugs may encourage even more impulses to utilize the fast accessory pathway connection, producing clinical deterioration. Vagotonic maneuvers, digoxin, verapamil, and adenosine are contraindicated. The pharmacological approach is to attack the accessory

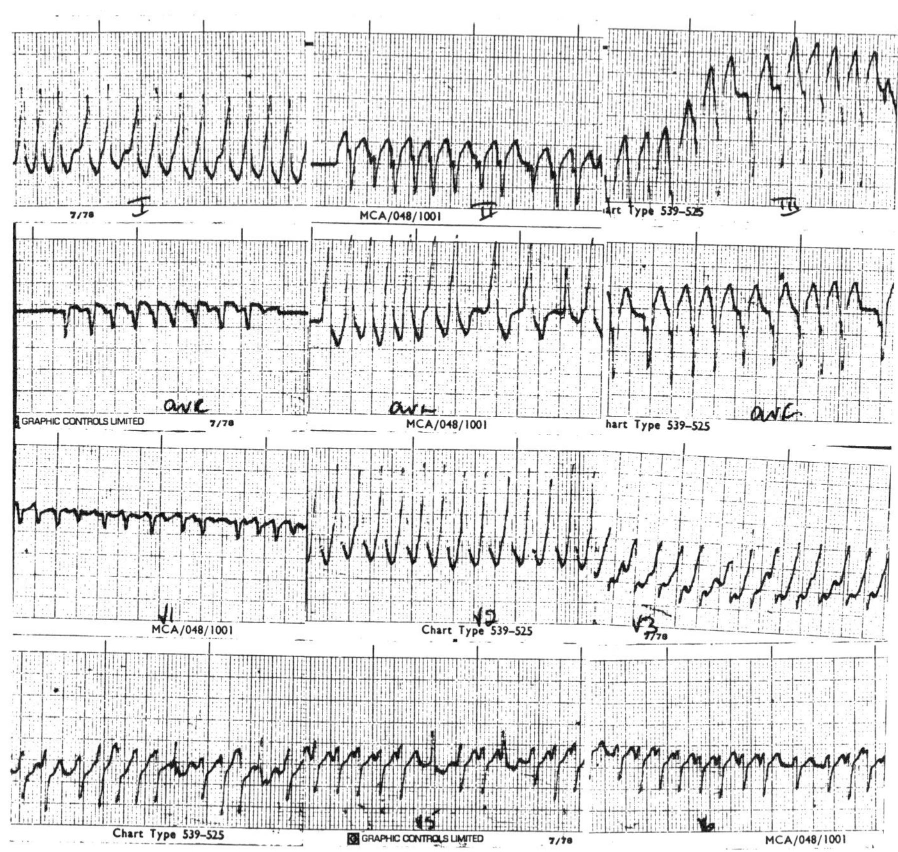

Figure 11: 12-lead ECG of AF complicating Wolff-Parkinson-White syndrome. The rapid atrial impulses are conducted over the accessory pathway to the ventricles. They produce a broad QRS that shows morphology variations. The resulting ventricular response rate is very rapid: 280 beats per minute. 30 seconds after this recording, the patient developed VF.

pathway. The best agents are the class 1c drugs propafenone and flecainide, the class 1a drug procainamide, and possibly amiodarone. In an acute crisis, early use of DC cardioversion is recommended.

CHRONIC PROPHYLAXIS

In the past, high-risk patients with accessory pathways, i.e.,. those with the capability of rapid atrioventricular transmission, were subjected to intensive electrophysiological research to identify drugs that favorably altered the electrophysiology of the accessory pathway. While chronic drug management is possible, it has many detractions. Relatively high plasma concentrations may be necessary to block or reduce function in the accessory pathway, bringing risks of toxicity. Plasma concentrations must be maintained at an effective level over 24 hours, perhaps necessitating frequent dosing intervals. In the event of intercurrent illness, particularly gastrointestinal disorders, absorption and metabolism of the drug may be modified and protection lost. For all these reasons, RF ablation has become the management of first choice for patients with high-risk accessory pathways. Any patient with known WPW syndrome (i.e., with an antegradely functioning accessory pathway) who has been syncopal or has had documented atrial fibrillation with short RR intervals (less than 220 ms) or rapid reciprocating tachycardias (cycle lengths 280 ms or less) should be considered to be at high risk and investigated and managed by RF ablation as necessary.

THE ASYMPTOMATIC INDIVIDUAL

The dramatic advances in management of accessory pathway arrhythmias is creating pressure to characterize the electrophysiology of all known accessory pathways. Many authorities recommend that with ECG evidence of pre-excitation in even an asymptomatic individual, investigation and therapy (if necessary) should be offered. The rationale is that the first symptom for some patients is sudden death. No intervention, however, is entirely innocuous. Despite the attractions of RF ablation, morbidity and mortality rarely occur. The younger the patient, the more persuasive is the argument to investigate. In general, problematic arrhythmias occur in the teens and early 20s. Individuals found to have antegradely functioning accessory pathways in their late 20s and older are less likely to have high-risk pathways. A case can therefore be made for relatively aggressive investigation of young individuals.

PEDIATRIC PRACTICE

Accessory pathways are a congenital abnormality. Reciprocating tachycardia is a problem in the first year of life, when it may present as cardiac failure or difficulties with feeding. Traditionally, digoxin has been used to control the arrhythmia, and in this setting it is an acceptable therapy. In infants and young children, the electrophysiology of the AV node is not dissimilar to that of the accessory pathway, and it probably matters little which of the two structures is targeted. Moreover, in the first year of life, the relatively small size of the atria all but precludes the development of atrial fibrillation. Typically, after the first year of life accessory pathways produce few problems, but at the onset of puberty arrhythmias may recur. This may be because of changes in the electrophysiology of the AV node. There is evidence that digoxin is detrimental in older children and adults with WPW syndrome. The drug may encourage the development of atrial fibrillation and may facilitate conduction over the accessory pathway. For this reason, digoxin therapy used for accessory pathway arrhythmias in young children should be reviewed as the child ages and should not be continued beyond the age of 8 years unless by recommendation of a specialist.

Para Atrioventricular Nodal Reentry Tachycardias

Half of all sustained narrow QRS tachycardias are due to a reentrant mechanism involving the AV node and juxta nodal atrial myocardium. This arrhythmia has been extensively investigated.

ANATOMY

The actual physical structures that support the arrhythmia are not as well established as the muscular atrioventricular connections involved in the Wolff-Parkinson-White syndrome. It seems likely, however, that atrial inputs to the lower reaches of the AV node may be a crucial part of the circuit (22).

ELECTROCARDIOGRAM

Para AV nodal reentry tachycardia produces a narrow QRS complex. The tachycardia cycle length is typically around 300 ms (200 beats per minute). P waves are usually not visible because they occur at the same time as the QRS complex (Figure 12).

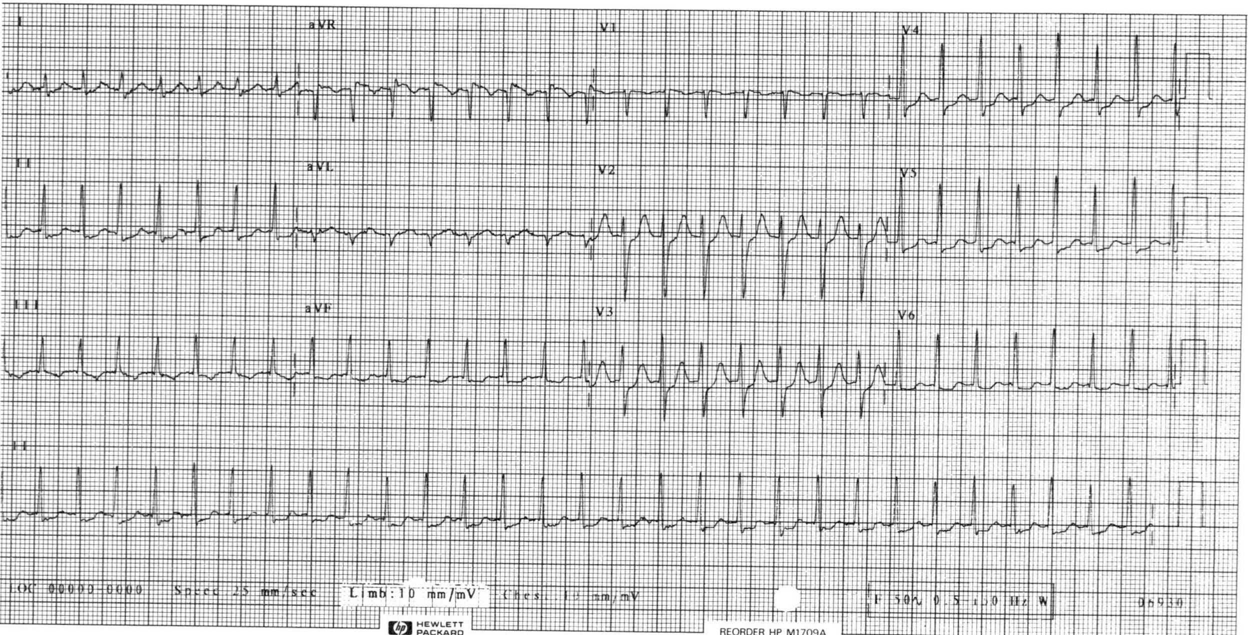

Figure 12: 12-lead ECG of para AV nodal reentry tachycardia. The rate is 180 beats per minute. The P waves are hidden within the QRS complexes.

ACUTE TERMINATION

Since AV nodal structures are pivotally involved in this arrhythmia, it is not surprising that acute termination may be accomplished by vagotonic maneuvers including Valsalva, the diving reflex, and carotid sinus massage. In the past, intravenous verapamil was recommended for termination. Although there is no contraindication to its use for this purpose, and despite its efficacy, in many countries adenosine has replaced verapamil. This strategy is designed to avoid the hazards of verapamil if wrongly administered to patients with VT.

CHRONIC PROPHYLAXIS

Para AV nodal reentry tachycardia is uncommon before the teenage years. The peak age of its presentation lies between 18 and 30 years. Affected patients have an anatomical mechanism for the arrhythmia, and it is usual for them to suffer repetitive attacks. Long-term prophylaxis may be achieved by a variety of drugs. Unlike Wolff-Parkinson-White syndrome, in this condition there is no bypass of the ventricular rate-limiting properties of the AV node and there is no risk of ventricular fibrillation if the patient develops atrial fibrillation. Digoxin has been the favored drug for management of this arrhythmia and it is moderately effective. It affects the AV nodal limb of the circuit. Often, relatively high doses are required for efficacy, and not uncommonly verapamil or diltiazem may be added. Verapamil and diltiazem may also be used as individual therapies. Despite the prevalence of para AV nodal reentry tachycardia, its drug susceptibility has not been as well established as that for accessory pathway arrhythmias. In some patients, para AV nodal reentry tachycardia is critically dependent on a specific setting of autonomic tone. In these patients, a beta-blocker may be useful. Management may also target the atrial inputs to the AV node, in which case class 1c drugs such as propafenone and flecainide and the class 3 drug amiodarone may be tried.

In the past, invasive electrophysiological procedures were performed to diagnose this particular form of narrow QRS reentry tachycardia. It is characterized by a so-called discontinuous AV nodal curve or a "jump" in the AV nodal curve (Figure 13). This feature signifies that there are two conduction routes either from atria to ventricles or from ventricles to atria.

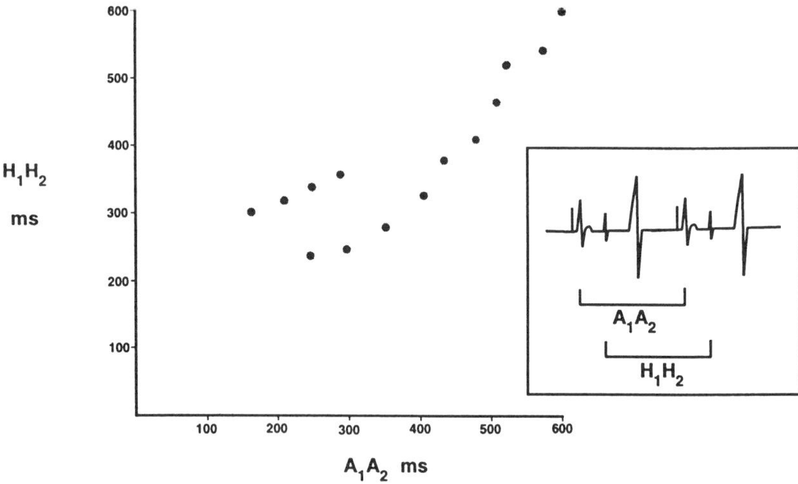

Figure 13: AV nodal curve demonstrating the so-called "jump" in antegrade AV nodal transmission. The plot is calculated by measuring A_1A_2 and H_1H_2 intervals from extrastimulus testing, as shown in the inset.

It was formerly considered a specific finding, but recent investigations reveal that so-called dual AV nodal physiology may be found in patients who have never had arrhythmias.

NONPHARMACOLOGICAL THERAPY

For years it was thought that the para AV nodal reentry tachycardia circuit was contained within the AV node. With the realization that an extra nodal structure was involved, a surgical approach was developed and thereafter nonpharmacological techniques were explored. Because the surgical techniques meant working very close to the AV node, there was a risk of producing complete AV block. While undesirable, this would cure the arrhythmias—but it left the patient dependent on a pacemaker. Surgery for this arrhythmia has been abandoned in favor of RF ablation.

RF catheter ablation has an important role in the management of para AV nodal reentry tachycardia. Either the fast antegrade or the slow retrograde pathway may be targeted. Since the fast antegrade pathway lies within the AV node itself there is a considerable risk (up to 5%) of producing complete heart block if this approach is used. Targeting the slow retrograde pathway provides a 95% or better chance of successful cure with a less than 1% risk of AV nodal damage requiring pacing (23). The fact that such a procedure has become almost routine in major electrophysiological centers is a testimony to the pace of research in understanding the mechanism and anatomy of arrhythmias.

CHAPTER 7

"True" Atrial Tachycardia and Other Rare Atrial Arrhythmias

"True" atrial tachycardia accounts for no more than 5% of all narrow QRS tachycardias. It can arise in either atria and may be either automatic or reentrant. The arrhythmia may be particularly persistent. P waves (their morphology depends on the location of the atrial generator) precede narrow QRS complexes (Figure 14). Occasionally multiple arrhythmia generators are present, giving rise to an appearance labeled chaotic or multifocal atrial tachycardia. The latter arrhythmia often eventually degenerates to atrial fibrillation

True atrial tachycardias are often associated with structural heart disease in which there are atrial abnormalities.

ACUTE TERMINATION

Acute termination of true atrial tachycardia is difficult. Efforts to alter AV nodal electrophysiology will merely temporarily slow the ventricular response rate but will do nothing to terminate the fundamental arrhythmogenic process. Even synchronized DC conversion may be rewarded by only a brief period of sinus rhythm before the arrhythmia restarts. True atrial tachycardias are among the most recalcitrant of all arrhythmias. Powerful antiarrhythmic interventions with the class 1c drugs propafenone and

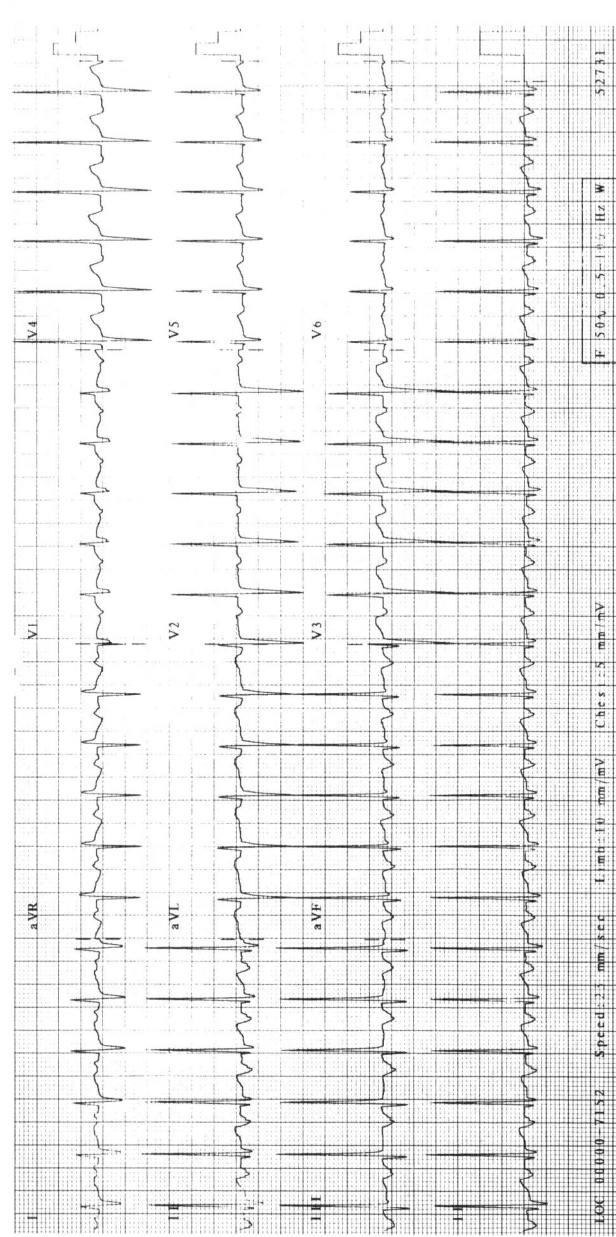

Figure 14: 12-lead ECG of "true" atrial tachycardia. Tall positive P waves are seen in V1. Their rate is 150 beats per minute. There is a variable ventricular rate averaging 90 beats per minute. This was a low medial right atrial tachycardia.

flecainide or with the class 3 drug amiodarone are often necessary, but even they may fail to restore sinus rhythm.

CHRONIC PROPHYLAXIS

Any factors considered relevant in causing the arrhythmia should be addressed. For instance, reduction of atrial wall tension—by whatever means—may be useful, as would correction of electrolyte abnormalities. The persistent nature of true atrial tachycardias brings a threat of tachycardia-related cardiomyopathy to affected patients. This condition is probably frequently missed but should be considered in any patient presenting with an unexplained cardiomyopathy and a heart rate above 120 beats per minute. In resistant forms of true atrial tachycardia, nonpharmacological therapy has an important role. At cardiac surgery, the arrhythmogenic generator can be mapped and extirpated. Increasingly, however, RF ablation is being used for management. Intra-atrial catheters perform the mapping, with an RF lesion or lesions being delivered by a specially designed large-tip ablation catheter. Complications are rare, and serious complications even rarer. Success rates of over 90% are routinely being achieved (24).

CHAPTER 8

Ventricular Ectopic Beats

Of all the clinical arrhythmias, ventricular ectopic beats create the most anxiety, have the least immediate impact, and are the most likely ECG phenomena to trigger inappropriate prescription of therapy.

Ventricular ectopic beats are commonplace. Even young normal individuals may demonstrate occasional ectopic beats on 24-hour ECGs. Unquestionably, however, ventricular ectopic beat rates rise in the presence of cardiac disease, particularly cardiac disease that has an impact on ventricular muscle. Ischemic heart disease is far and away the most important etiological basis of ventricular ectopic beats.

SYMPTOMATOLOGY

Ventricular ectopic beats are very variably perceived by those affected. Many are completely unappreciated. Some individuals may have many hundreds of ventricular ectopic beats and be completely unaware of any perturbation of their cardiac rhythm. In contrast, some particularly sensitive individuals are seriously disturbed by a single ventricular ectopic beat.

Even a single ventricular ectopic beat has some hemodynamic impact. Coming earlier than expected in the cardiac cycle and activating the ventricle without the benefit of the His-Purkinje system, cardiac output associated with that beat will be lower than normal. There is usually a compensatory pause in which the ventricle overfills with an augmented stroke volume on the next normal beat. Many patients who are aware of ventricular ectopic beats perceive the augmented sinus beat rather than the arrhythmic beat itself.

PATTERNS

Ventricular ectopic beats may occur in many patterns. In the past it was fashionable to classify them according to the Lown classification (25), but this no longer has clinical relevance. Ventricular ectopic beats that occur in salvos are probably best considered variants of ventricular tachycardia (see later). Ventricular ectopic beats of different shapes are described as multiform. At least a proportion represent two or more different ectopic generator sites. It has been suggested that this might have prognostic significance; indeed, some studies have provided such evidence. The data are not consistent, and any additional risk of a multiform pattern, if it exists, is small. R-on-T ventricular ectopic beats fall on the T wave of the preceding sinus beat (Figure 15). An indication of inhomogeneity of repolarization, they are a dramatic demonstration that myocardium can be restimulated at a time when much of the ventricular muscle has not repolarized. The propagated ectopic beat further increases the dispersion. R-on-T ectopic beats are not unique to the acute phase of myocardial infarction (MI) but are seen most often in that setting. Many episodes of ventricular fibrillation that

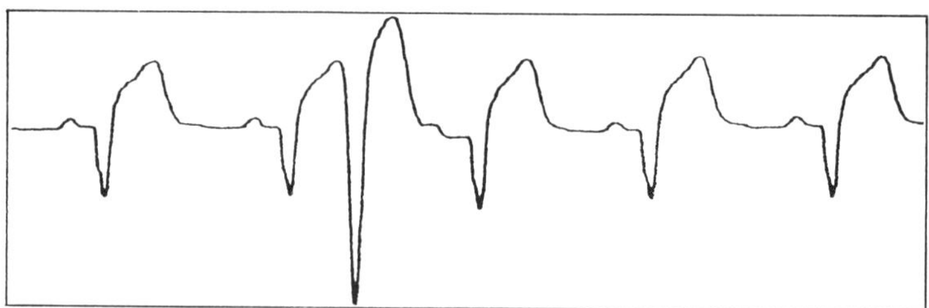

Figure 15:　　An R-on-T ventricular ectopic beat recorded from a monitor lead. The patient was in the acute phase of myocardial infarction.

occur in the acute phase of myocardial infarction arise from R-on-T ectopic beats. In the past it was held that R-on-T ectopic beats might predict the occurrence of ventricular fibrillation, but this is now known not to be the case. Most R-on-T ectopic beats pass without consequence. Their appearance is an important indicator that the threshold for ventricular fibrillation is lowered.

TREATMENT: SYMPTOMS

The hemodynamic upset of ventricular ectopic beats is an insufficient reason to require their acute suppression. Most management of ventricular ectopic beats is directed at chronic control. The aim of therapy is to control symptoms and/or improve prognosis. Symptom control may be achieved by modest changes in ventricular ectopic beat patterns. Prolonging the coupling interval or reducing the frequency of events may be sufficient to achieve a satisfactory clinical outcome. Very many antiarrhythmic drugs have actions against ventricular ectopic beats. They include all the class 1 antiarrhythmic agents such as the 1a therapies quinidine, procainamide, and disopyramide; the 1b agents lignocaine and mexiletine; and the class 1c drugs propafenone and flecainide. Ventricular ectopic beats are often rate-related, and in some patients beta-blockers may offer good control. Beta-blockers should be considered first-line therapy in patients with ischemic heart disease because they bring additional anti-ischemic benefits. The class 3 drug amiodarone can also suppress ventricular ectopic beats, but its noncardiac toxicity renders it less attractive for use in patients in whom only symptom control is neccessary.

TREATMENT: PROGNOSIS

Ventricular ectopic beats are associated with an adverse prognosis in a wide range of cardiovascular diseases. Depending on pattern and frequency, ventricular ectopic beats are associated with an up to threefold increase in mortality in survivors of myocardial infarction compared with those whose late infarct course is not as complicated (27). Ventricular ectopic beats also have prognostic significance in such diverse conditions as aortic stenosis (28) and dilated cardiomyopathy (29). The aim in treating prognostically relevant ventricular ectopic beats must be to improve prognosis. Suppression of ventricular ectopic beats in infarct survivors has not been rewarded by patient benefit. Trials involving class 1 drugs such as flecainide (2), encainide (2), moricizine (30), and mexiletine (31) have achieved arrhythmia suppression but in some cases have produced a statistically significant increase in mortality (32). A study with the experimental antiarrhythmic drug d-sotalol (a class 3 antiarrhythmic drug) has also been associated with an increase in mortality. These findings have caused concern and created some confusion. Powerful antiarrhythmic drugs can bring unwanted effects. Many of the agents depress left ventricular performance, and almost every antiarrhythmic drug is capable of aggravating arrhythmias or creating new ones, a process called proarrhythmia or arrhythmogenesis. Most ventricular ectopic beats add only modestly to prognosis postinfarction, and many reported studies included relatively low-risk patients. There was little opportunity for these drugs to show benefit since the follow-up mortality in the placebo-treated patients in these trials was already very low. It was much easier, as happened, to show detrimental effects of the drugs.

The clear message is that ventricular ectopic beats indicate patients with cardiovascular disease who are at higher risk than similar patients without the arrhythmia. The therapeutic approach must be to ameliorate the underlying disease and recognize that the ventricular ectopic beats are merely a marker.

VENTRICULAR ECTOPIC BEATS IN APPARENTLY NORMAL INDIVIDUALS

There is a continuing controversy about the significance of ventricular ectopic beats in apparently normal individuals. The evidence is contradictory but would support the suggestion that a prognostic implication becomes apparent only when the apparently normal individual has more than 200 such beats per hour or has a lower frequency of arrhythmias but in the presence of structural cardiac disease (33). With increasing use of medical examinations for employment, health screening, and insurance, more individuals with ventricular ectopic beats are being detected. On detection, the individual should be reassured. The probability is very great that the finding is of no immediate or late prognostic significance. A detailed history and physical examination should be obtained and steps taken to exclude the presence of underlying structural heart disease. As a minimum, this involves a 12-lead electrocardiogram and an echocardiogram, but exercise testing and nuclear or MRI imaging may also be necessary. Only in exceptional circumstances will invasive investigations be necessary. These should not be undertaken lightly and without due consideration of the benefits and risks they may have for the patient.

Ischemic Ventricular Tachycardia

Ventricular arrhythmias are a common accompaniment of ischemic heart disease. Ventricular ectopic beats may occur during angina pectoris, and in Prinzmetal variant angina, in which myocardial ischemia is caused by coronary artery spasm (34), salvos of ectopic beats and ventricular tachycardia are a characteristic feature.

ACUTE MYOCARDIAL INFARCTION VENTRICULAR TACHYCARDIA

It is during the acute phase of myocardial infarction, at a time when there is dense myocardial ischemia but before myocardial necrosis, that ventricular arrhythmias are most common. As has already been discussed, a variety of patterns of ventricular ectopic beats occur at this time. Ventricular tachycardia is defined as three or more consecutive ventricular ectopic beats at a rate equal to or greater than 120 beats per minute. It is common in the first 24 hours of infarction, but the arrhythmia is characteristically short-lived and often polymorphic (Figure 16) (26). The rate is usually irregular. These features suggest an automatic basis for the arrhythmia, which is consistent with the disappearance of this arrhythmic event as myocardial necrosis occurs.

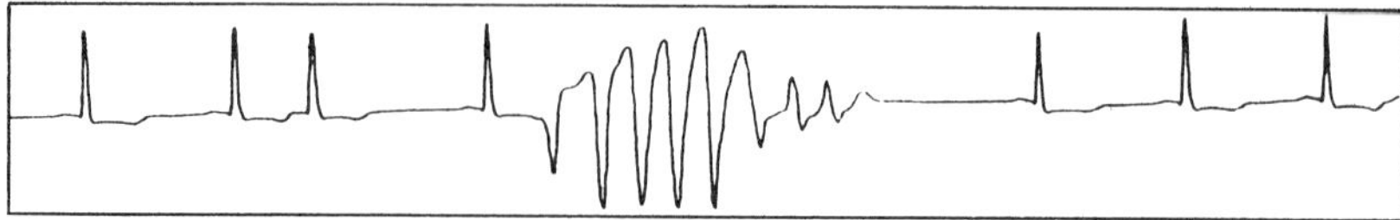

Figure 16:   Monitor lead recording of a typical brief polymorphic burst of VT during acute-phase myocardial infarction.

POST-MYOCARDIAL-INFARCTION
VENTRICULAR TACHYCARDIA

In up to 10% of infarct survivors, ventricular tachycardia is a late complication. In contradistinction to the pattern seen during acute ischemia, whether associated with angina or early-phase infarction, this ventricular tachycardia is usually stable, monomorphic, regular, and persistent (Figure 17) (35). These features suggest a reentrant mechanism, and this has been confirmed by programmed electrical stimulation using intracardiac catheters. In affected patients, critically timed stimuli can provoke ventricular tachycardia. Similarly critically timed stimuli can stop the arrhythmia. Cardiac mapping has provided the final confirmation of the macro-reentrant nature of postinfarction ventricular tachycardia.

Postinfarction VT is a dangerous arrhythmia. Patients who have suffered myocardial damage are particularly vulnerable to the consequences of this arrhythmia because during the event there may be inadequate time

Figure 17:   12-lead ECG of a sustained monomorphic VT (ventricular rate 200 beats per minute). The QRS is broad: approximately 180 ms. Note that the QRS is predominantly negative in all the V leads, a feature strongly associated with a diagnosis of VT. The patient had sustained a myocardial infarction 3 months previously. P waves are not seen clearly but are probably present; they are responsible for the subtle variations seen in the ST segments of the V leads.

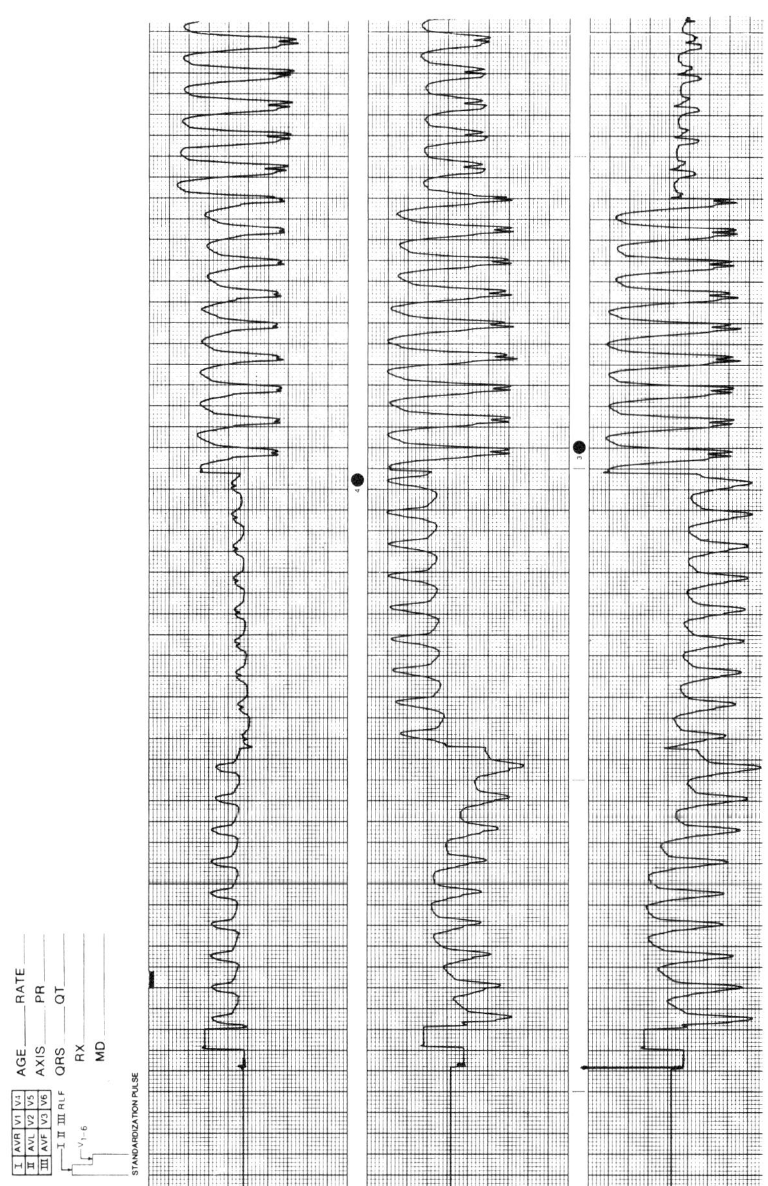

for ventricular filling and, worse, jeopardy of the important diastolic period during which coronary artery blood flow occurs. Although some patients are almost unaware of their ventricular tachycardia, most have important symptoms. Many suffer hemodynamic collapse, and in a few the arrhythmia quickly deteriorates to ventricular fibrillation.

The electrocardiographic appearance is of a broad QRS tachycardia (QRS 120 ms). The broader the QRS, the more likely is the diagnosis that it is ventricular tachycardia. Any broad QRS tachycardia in the setting of ischemic heart disease is ventricular tachycardia until proven otherwise. Further confirmation of the diagnosis may be obtained by the finding of dissociated P waves and/or the presence of capture beats which occur when a P wave fortuitously occurs at a time when it can be conducted through the AV node to capture the ventricle just ahead of the tachycardia generator. The resultant QRS is a mixture of the QRS that might have been produced by exclusive AV nodal–His-Purkinje conduction and that produced by the tachycardia.

Acute treatment: drug therapy

Sustained monomorphic VT postinfarction requires urgent treatment. In some patients it is a real emergency, as when there is hemodynamic collapse. Termination of established monomorphic VT may be accomplished by either drug or electrical therapy. If the affected patient is not in extremis, blood pressure is acceptable, and the patient is conscious and responding, intravenous administration of 100 mg lignocaine is appropriate. If this drug has no effect and stable circumstances still pertain, the dose may be cautiously repeated 5 minutes later.

Acute treatment: electrical therapy

In the event that lignocaine does not work or that the patient has collapsed, a synchronized DC shock should be first-line therapy. The defibrillator should be synchronized to the R wave of the tachycardia. An inappropriately timed discharge will often provoke ventricular fibrillation. In that unfortunate event, a second defibrillating DC shock would have to be delivered. Postinfarction sustained VT is an electrically organized arrhythmia, and restoration of sinus rhythm may be achieved with relatively low energy levels. Fifty Joules may be sufficient to terminate the event but if this is not successful, there should be a quick progression through the defibrillator energy levels until termination is achieved. Even 30 Joules of electrical energy is painful for patients and general anesthesia is a necessity.

Posttermination: drug therapy

The appearance of sustained monomorphic postinfarction VT is an indicator that the anatomical substrate for this arrhythmia has been established by the infarct and/or the subsequent myocardial repair process. This means that the patient has a chronic risk of arrhythmia recurrence. Because of the danger posed by the arrhythmia, it is appropriate to consider prophylactic therapy. Empirical drug therapy may be chosen. Amiodarone is the drug of choice for this approach because, of all the antiarrhythmic drugs, it offers the best efficacy (36). Its drawbacks of noncardiac unwanted effects are important but in the context of the risk posed by the arrhythmia these risks are often acceptable. Nonetheless, every effort should be made to use the lowest dose consistent with successful arrhythmia prophylaxis.

Since the arrhythmia can be provoked by programmed stimulation, this technique offers a possibility of selecting a drug that may not have the disadvantages of amiodarone. Several studies have shown that when a drug renders the arrhythmia incapable of reinitiation by programmed stimulation, that therapy will be associated with an improved prognosis (37). Drugs that may be tested include the class 1 agents. Programmed electrical stimulation is less reliable in the assessment of beta-blockers and amiodarone. Of the class 1 agents, propafenone and flecainide are perhaps the most powerful in preventing postinfarction VT. The untoward results obtained with class 1c therapy in the Cardiac Arrhythmia Suppression Trials (2,30) have prompted many to abandon the use of these agents in patients with ischemic heart disease. There is certainly every evidence that such therapy should not be used in postinfarction patients with ventricular ectopic beats in attempts to improve prognosis but the situation is different in patients with manifest ventricular tachycardia. Their VT is a serious risk; for them, effective class 1c therapy—i.e.,. therapy that prevents VT—may be acceptable. In this specific situation, the benefit of these drugs can outweigh their risks.

Posttermination: nonpharmacological therapy

Even with an extensive search for effective therapy, only about 60% of patients have their arrhythmia controlled by antiarrhythmic drugs. For the remainder, nonpharmacological therapy may have a role.

Map-directed VT surgery is possible (38). The arrhythmia generator or vulnerable parts of its circuit can be identified during the operation by mapping. Surgical removal of these areas will control the arrhythmia. The surgery is substantial, and, although curative and offering a success rate of 90% or better, depending on patient selection, there may be an operative mortality ranging from 3 to 20%. Patients with an anterior infarct, an aneurysm, or single-vessel disease who have no valvular dysfunction and are not in heart failure are, not surprisingly, good-risk patients. Those in heart failure or with inferior infarcts or mitral regurgitation carry the highest operative risk.

An alternative to surgery is the implantable cardioverter defibrillator (ICD) (39). In the past this option was unattractive because it entailed the delivery of high-energy shocks to patients who were conscious but experiencing VT. New developments in the ICD have enabled antitachycardia pacing. Over 95% of patients with ischemic VT will respond to this pacing modality. In the event that the pacing provokes ventricular fibrillation, the implanted device can deliver a lifesaving high-energy shock. Were it not for the cost of these units and, to some extent, the complexity of their programming, they would have a wider application.

A final possibility for nonpharmacological management is radiofrequency energy to destroy the generator site. Although theoretically possible, with a few successful case reports in the literature, for the present this approach must remain experimental (40). There are many cogent reasons that this technique would not be expected to be applicable to more than a very small minority of affected patients.

Nonischemic Ventricular Tachycardia

Ventricular tachycardia may complicate a variety of types of cardiovascular disease. While it is most common in association with ischemic heart disease, VT occurs in other situations.

RIGHT VENTRICULAR DYSPLASIA

Right ventricular dysplasia is an ill-understood condition in which the myocardium of the right ventricle is progressively replaced by fatty tissue (41). Evidence now suggests that it is not exclusively confined to the right ventricle but that in many patients septal and left ventricular involvement also occurs. In most patients, however, left ventricular function is relatively normal and affected patients may tolerate their episodes of ventricular tachycardia surprisingly well. The ECG shows typical appearances of ventricular tachycardia with a broad QRS complex and, in some, dissociated P waves and/or fusion complexes. Because this arrhythmia arises from reentrant activity in the right ventricle, a left bundle branch block configuration is commonly seen. As the condition can have an extensive effect in the right ventricle, multiple types of ventricular tachycardia may occur. The unusual left bundle branch block configuration of the arrhythmia (Figure 18) and the appearance of T-wave inversion in V1–V3 on the surface ECG in sinus rhythm are strong clues to the diagnosis. Therapy is directed at preventing

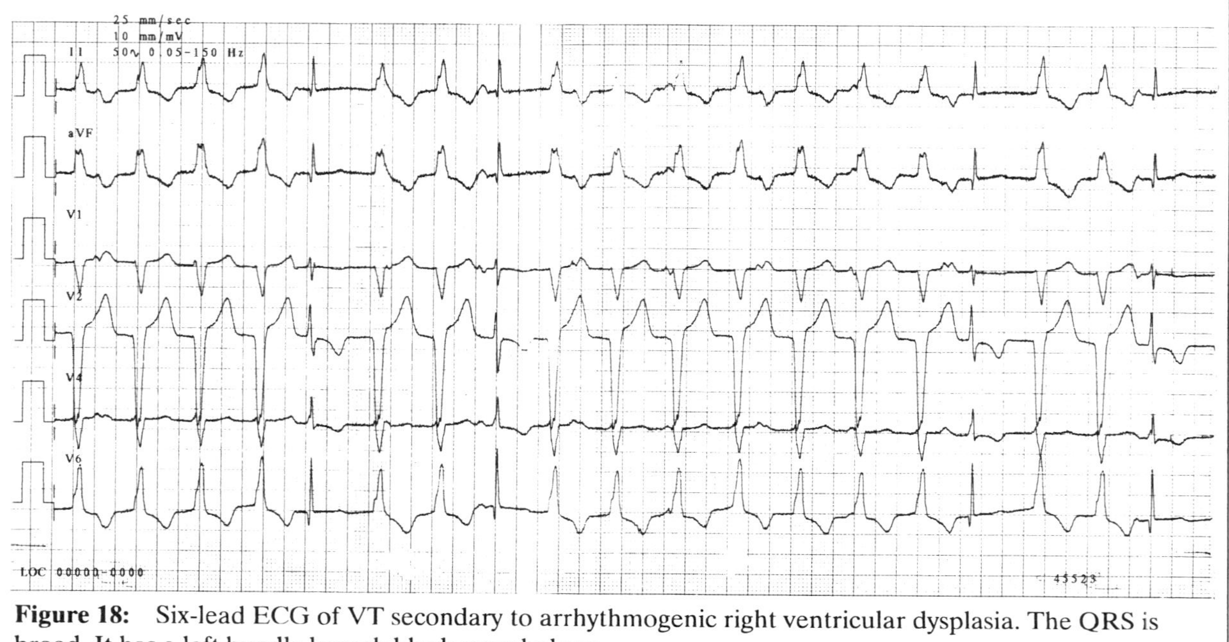

Figure 18: Six-lead ECG of VT secondary to arrhythmogenic right ventricular dysplasia. The QRS is broad. It has a left bundle branch block morphology.

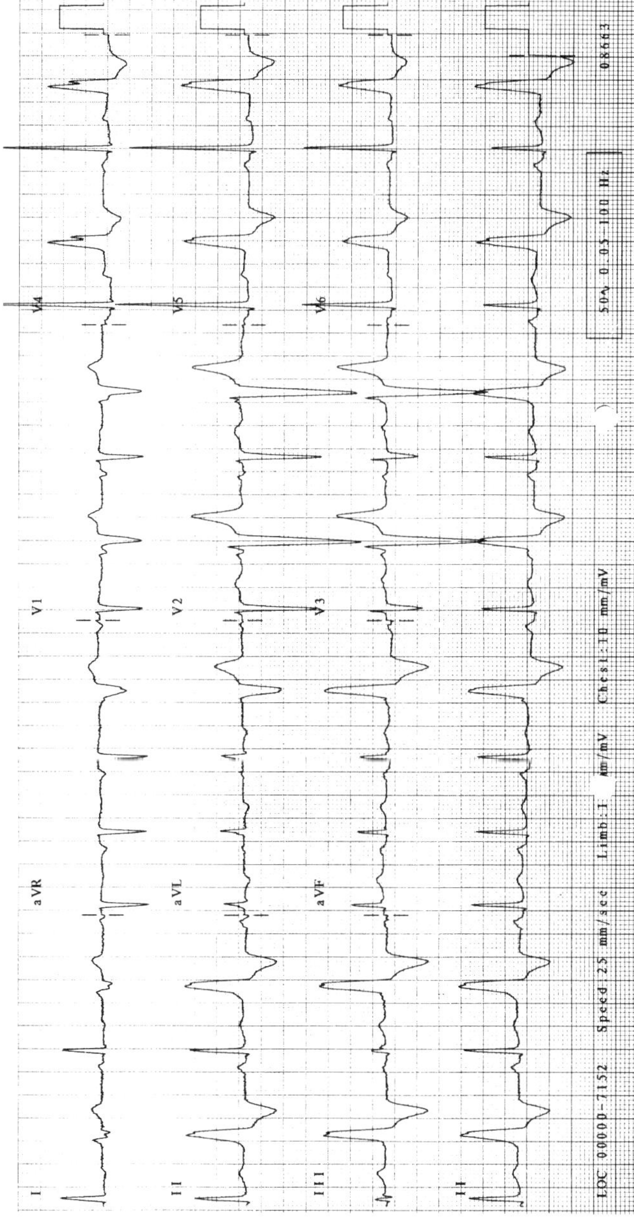

Figure 19: 12-lead ECG of patient with RV outflow tract tachycardia. This shows a typical appearance when not in sustained tachycardia. There are coupled ventricular ectopic beats with a left bundle branch block morphology and a frontal axis of +90°.

events. Effective interventions include the class 1c drugs propafenone and flecainide, the 1b drug mexiletine, and amiodarone.

RIGHT VENTRICULAR OUTFLOW TRACT TACHYCARDIA

Right ventricular outflow tract tachycardia affects young, apparently healthy individuals (42). The arrhythmia is catecholamine-dependent and as such is often provoked by exercise. The arrhythmia is often very well tolerated, but as attacks become more frequent or in circumstances in which the arrhythmia is very rapid, disabling symptoms may be present. The ECG pattern of the arrhythmia is of the left bundle branch block configuration VT with a vertical ($+90°$) axis (Figure 19).

In a few patients, therapy with beta-blockers is effective, but in young individuals achieving full protective beta-blockade is difficult and often associated with unacceptable unwanted effects such as tiredness. The arrhythmia is probably due to an automatic generator situated in the right ventricular outflow tract. Remarkable successes are now being achieved with radiofrequency ablation of this arrhythmia. In the event of failure of beta-blockade or nontolerance of that therapy, early recourse to RF ablation is appropriate. This has the attraction of offering a cure (95% success rates) with relatively few risks (43).

OTHER CONDITIONS

Ventricular tachycardia can complicate a wide variety of other cardiovascular conditions including mitral valve prolapse, aortic stenosis, dilated cardiomyopathies, and hypertrophic cardiomyopathy. In all these circumstances the arrhythmia is often short-lived, polymorphic, and irregular. This suggests an automatic basis for the arrhythmia. In many situations the arrhythmia may be provoked or aggravated by catecholamines. Not surprisingly, then, beta-blockers have a role to play in some situations, for example, in mitral valve prolapse and hypertrophic cardiomyopathy. In the latter circumstance, however, some authorities would hold that amiodarone is the drug of choice for managing VT detected in patients with hypertrophic cardiomyopathy (44).

VT complicating cardiac disease has prognostic implication. The untoward consequences associated with the arrhythmia may arise directly because of the arrhythmia, in which case arrhythmia control will be rewarded by benefits for the patient. In other circumstances—for instance, perhaps, in dilated cardiomyopathy—the VT is merely a marker of a severe underlying problem. In such cases, suppression of the VT may not be rewarded by improved prognosis, and attention should be directed to the basic disease process.

CHAPTER 11

Torsade de Pointes

Torsade de pointes (twisting of the points) is a very important ventricular tachyarrhythmia. Since its description in 1966 (45), there has been great debate as to how specific the arrhythmia is and how it may be distinguished from polymorphic VT. Classically, torsade de pointes is a polymorphic VT that shows cyclical change of QRS vector (Figure 20). It generally arises in situations of bradycardia with QT prolongation. It is associated with the congenital long QT syndromes and with drug toxicity.

CONGENITAL LONG QT SYNDROMES

The congenital long QT syndromes are an important but rare cardiac problem (46). Affected individuals typically present in childhood or adolescence with syncopal attacks. The resting ECG is usually grossly abnormal, with marked QT prolongation and/or bizarre T-wave abnormalities. Syncopal events correspond with bursts of torsade de pointes. The genetic basis of the condition is now being unraveled. Several gene mutations can give rise to an appearance of long QT syndrome and torsade de pointes (47).

Treatment

The majority of the gene mutations involved in torsade de pointes create abnormalities of potassium channel behavior; in this group of patients, the

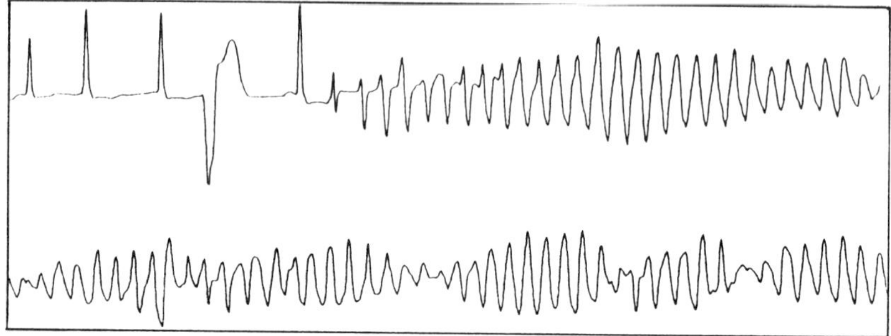

Figure 20:   Continuous monitor lead showing torsade de pointes.

best clinical successes have been achieved by prescription of beta-blockers (48). In the event of failure of that therapy, left stellate ganglionectomy and/or consideration of an implantable cardioverter defibrillator have been recommended. In a small but important proportion of children with long QT syndrome, the abnormality is based on the sodium channel. Early evidence might suggest a role for mexiletine therapy in controlling their problems.

DRUG-INDUCED LONG QT SYNDROME

It is well recognized that a variety of drugs may create arrhythmias: the phenomenon of proarrhythmia or drug arrhythmogenesis. The arrhythmia typically produced is torsade de pointes, and it is common that this arrhythmia is preceded by QT prolongation and/or T-wave abnormalities. The incriminated drugs include many antiarrhythmic drugs such as quinidine, flecainide, propafenone, sotalol, ibutilide, dofetilide, and, very rarely, amiodarone. Antibiotics, antidepressants, and antihistamines are just a few of the noncardiac medications that may also create this problem. Unexpected syncope occurring in a patient taking any medication should arouse suspicion. An ECG should be obtained. If the QT interval is abnormal, drug-related arrhythmogenesis should be strongly suspected.

Treatment

The management of drug-induced torsade de pointes has been debated. The generally agreed-on advice is to stop cardioactive medications, to normalize electrolytes (this may mean taking potassium and magnesium levels (49) to the upper part of the normal range), to rest the patient, and, if necessary, to consider cardiac pacing (preferably atrial) to counter bradycardia. Some have suggested active intervention to suppress ventricular tachycardia, but there is little evidence that this is useful or safe.

CHAPTER 12

Ventricular Fibrillation

Ventricular fibrillation (VF) is a lethal arrhythmia unless reversed by DC cardioversion. During ventricular fibrillation there is no coordinated ventricular contraction (Figure 21). Cardiac output ceases. Sinus rhythm can be restored in at least a proportion of patients by prompt global depolarization of the ventricular myocardium using either an external or internal defibrillator. There are anecdotal reports of pharmacological conversion of VF (50) to sinus rhythm, but there is no consistent evidence that this has a practical application.

Ventricular fibrillation is seen most commonly in the first 12 hours of acute myocardial infarction (26). At that time, if promptly dealt with, it has little or no prognostic implication. It is marginally more common in those with large infarcts and those with anterior infarcts than in those with small or inferior infarcts. It was once customary to give therapy to prevent VF, but this is now known not to be of value. Studies have shown that the incidence of VF can be reduced by prophylactic lignocaine administration to those in the earliest phase of infarction, but this therapy was associated with an increased risk of AV block, which effectively counterbalanced any anti-VF benefit (51).

Ventricular fibrillation also occurs as a terminal event. Although the electrocardiographic pattern is similar to that seen in the acute phase of infarction, restoration of sinus rhythm is rarely possible for VF associated with hypotension and heart failure.

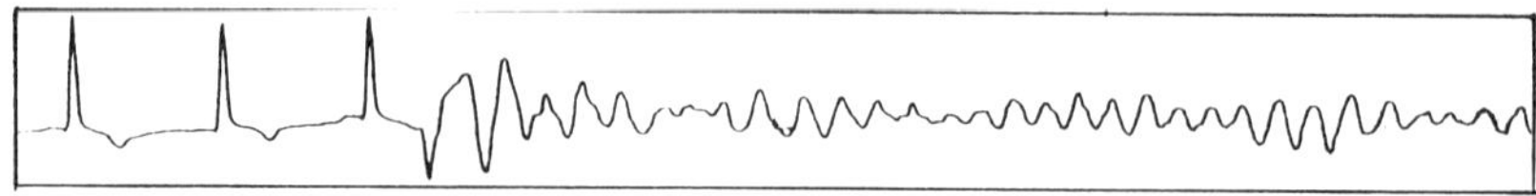

Figure 21: Monitor lead showing initiation of ventricular fibrillation.

ACUTE TREATMENT

When VF occurs, the circulation of blood is arrested, and within minutes irreversible brain damage may occur. Speedy treatment is essential. The arrhythmia produces an irregular baseline on the ECG, with no visible P waves or QRS complexes. A "chaotic" pattern is seen in which it is all but impossible to measure a rate. Based on crossings of the isoelectric line, the rate of ventricular fibrillation is in excess of 400 beats per minute. A high-energy DC shock is the only proven method of restoring sinus rhythm. Current international guidelines recommend an initial 200 Joule shock (52), followed, if unsuccessful, by a second 200 Joule shock. Only then is it recommended that a full-output (360–400 Joule) shock be given. It can be argued that in the setting of VF, where every second counts, there is little advantage in delivering less than the full output of the defibrillator for the first shock. Even modern defibrillators take time to recharge their capacitors in the event of a failed shock; this may jeopardize the patient's survival more than the shock-related myocardial damage. Ideally, shocks should be delivered through large-area electrodes with good gel contact and in an anteroposterior placement. If the first shock is unsuccessful, the defibrillator should be recharged and second, third, and fourth shocks delivered. There is some evidence that even an unsuccessful initial shock may reduce tissue impedance and improve the chances for restoring sinus rhythm with subsequent shocks. There have been many suggestions for additive therapies, such as epinephrine, bretylium, and lignocaine, to be used in the event of failure of DC shocks to restore sinus rhythm. None has been proved useful in humans.

Atrioventricular Block

The electrical link between the atria and the ventricles is crucial. It is over this link that modulated impulses generated by the sinus node enter the His-Purkinje network to initiate ventricular contraction.

NORMAL ATRIAL VENTRICULAR CONDUCTION

The delay in transit through the AV node varies according to heart rate and autonomic state. In this way the relationship between atrial and ventricular contraction is optimized. Conduction through the AV node is analyzed from the PR segment of the surface ECG. This ECG interval is not, however, entirely due to conduction time within the AV node. It includes intra-atrial conduction delay and the conduction time within the His-Purkinje network. The PR interval is measured from the onset of the P wave to the onset of the QRS complex. More detailed analysis of AV conduction is possible using intracardiac recordings of the His bundle potential which indicates activation of the His bundle. However, this investigation is rarely required for making either diagnosis or management decisions.

A normal PR interval is between 120 and 200—or, by some authorities, 220—ms. This is an arbitrary definition, as the PR interval varies with rate. Many fit young people with a normal resting sinus bradycardia will show PR prolongation of 240 or even 260 ms. In some circumstances, a

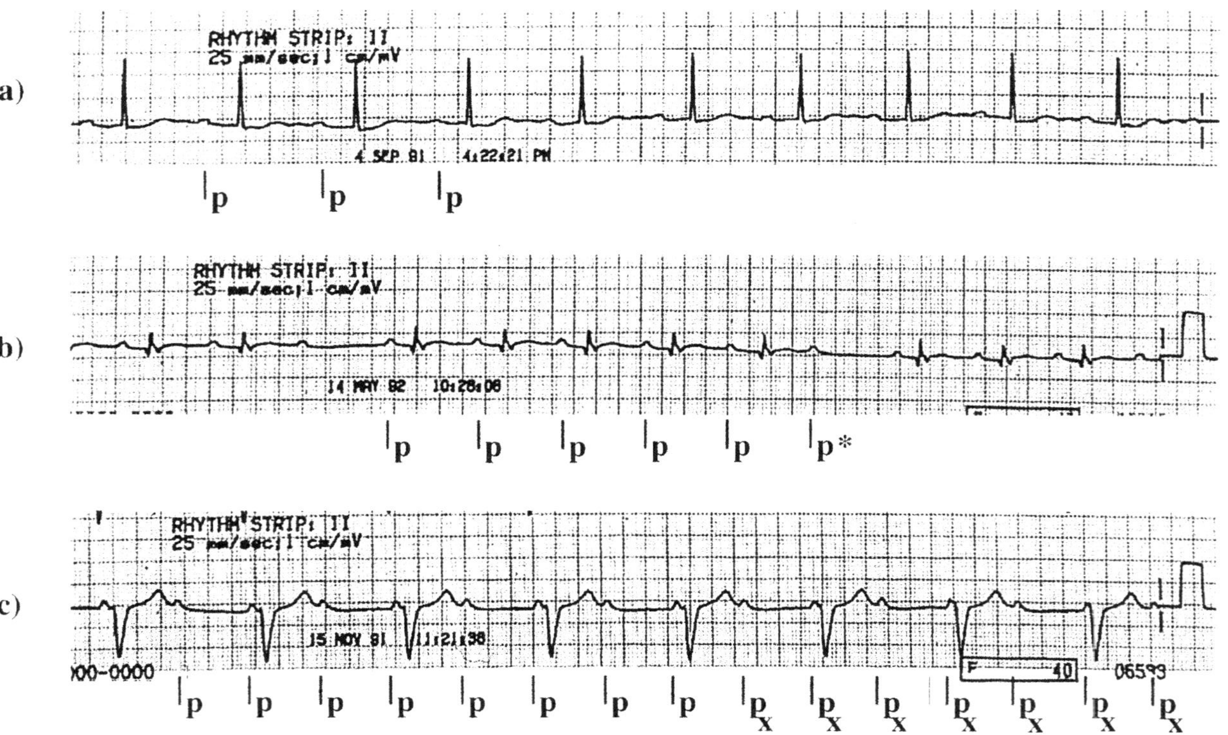

a)
RHYTHM STRIP: II
25 mm/sec; 1 cm/mV
4 SEP 81   4:22:21 PM
p   p   p

b)
RHYTHM STRIP: II
25 mm/sec; 1 cm/mV
14 MAY 82   10:28:06
p   p   p   p   p   p*

c)
RHYTHM STRIP: II
25 mm/sec; 1 cm/mV
15 NOV 81   11:21:38
000-0000
F   40   06593
p   p   p   p   p   p   p   p   px   px   px   px   px   px   px

"normal" PR interval of 180 ms may be abnormal, for instance, when the heart rate is 120 beats per minute or greater.

ATRIOVENTRICULAR BLOCK

AV block is the term used for a disturbance of atrioventricular conduction. Classically, three forms are described: first-, second-, and third-degree AV block (Figure 22).

First-degree AV block

In first-degree AV block, the PR interval is prolonged. The implication is that the transit time through the AV node is delayed. Sometimes the delay is in transatrial conduction. In first-degree AV block, each P wave is followed by a QRS complex (Figure 22a). First-degree heart block is common and not necessarily abnormal. It occurs in normal individuals, typically during sleep when there is a bradycardia. It may occur in the waking hours in those athletically trained. First-degree AV block may occur with extreme vagotonia. It may also be produced by drug therapy including digoxin.

There is no important hemodynamic disturbance associated with first-degree AV block, and most patients are completely unaware of its presence. Its relevance is in its association with autonomic tone and/or drug therapies. Its occurrence in patients with suspected cardiac diseases including sarcoidosis, indicate important cardiac involvement.

No specific treatment is warranted or appropriate.

Figure 22: Various degrees of AV block. (a) First-degree. Every P wave is followed by a normal QRS. PR interval 320 ms (normal 120–200 ms). (b) Wenckebach (2°). There is progressive PR prolongation until P* is blocked, with no resultant QRS. (c) Complete (3°). At first it appears that there is a 2:1 AV conduction (a form called high-grade 2° AV block). From Px, however, there is no association of P waves and the broad QRS complexes.

Second-degree AV block

In second-degree AV block, P waves are not always followed by QRS complexes. In one form, Wenckebach phenomenon, there is a progressive prolongation of the PR interval until a QRS is missed (Figure 22b). The cycle then restarts. In another form, Mobitz II, there is no prior PR prolongation; a QRS is missed, seemingly abruptly.

Second-degree AV block may rarely occur in normal individuals who are athletically trained. Most often, however, it is a pathological occurrence. It causes little or no immediate hemodynamic upset, although, because of the missed ventricular contraction, affected patients may notice palpitations. Its significance is its indication of important cardiovascular disease. It may be a harbinger of a more profound AV disturbance.

Most clinicians distinguish between Wenckebach and Mobitz II block, believing the former to be more benign than the latter. Recent studies have cast doubt on this and suggest that progression to complete AV block is relatively similar with either form (53). Second-degree AV block does not in itself warrant pacing, but in symptomatic patients or those with identified cardiac disease, prophylactic pacing may be appropriate.

A variant of second-degree AV block is so-called "high-grade block," in which there is a regular ratio between the P waves and QRS complexes: 2:1, 3:1, etc. This form of block is uncommon but it often progresses to complete AV block. It is seen most often in acute myocardial infarction.

Complete heart block

In complete heart block, no impulses are transmitted from the atria to the ventricles (Figure 22c). Were it not for the emergence of subsidiary pacemakers within the ventricular myocardium or the His-Purkinje system, death would occur. In many individuals, a slow idioventricular rhythm is established. This may be sufficient to maintain life, but its slow rate may cause cerebral dulling or even unconsciousness. Restoration of an adequate ventricular rate is essential and must be accomplished speedily. Ventricular pacing is the management of choice, but when complete heart block complicates inferior myocardial infarction, intravenous atropine may restore AV conduction without the need for permanent cardiac pacing. In contrast, when complete heart block complicates anterior infarction, permanent

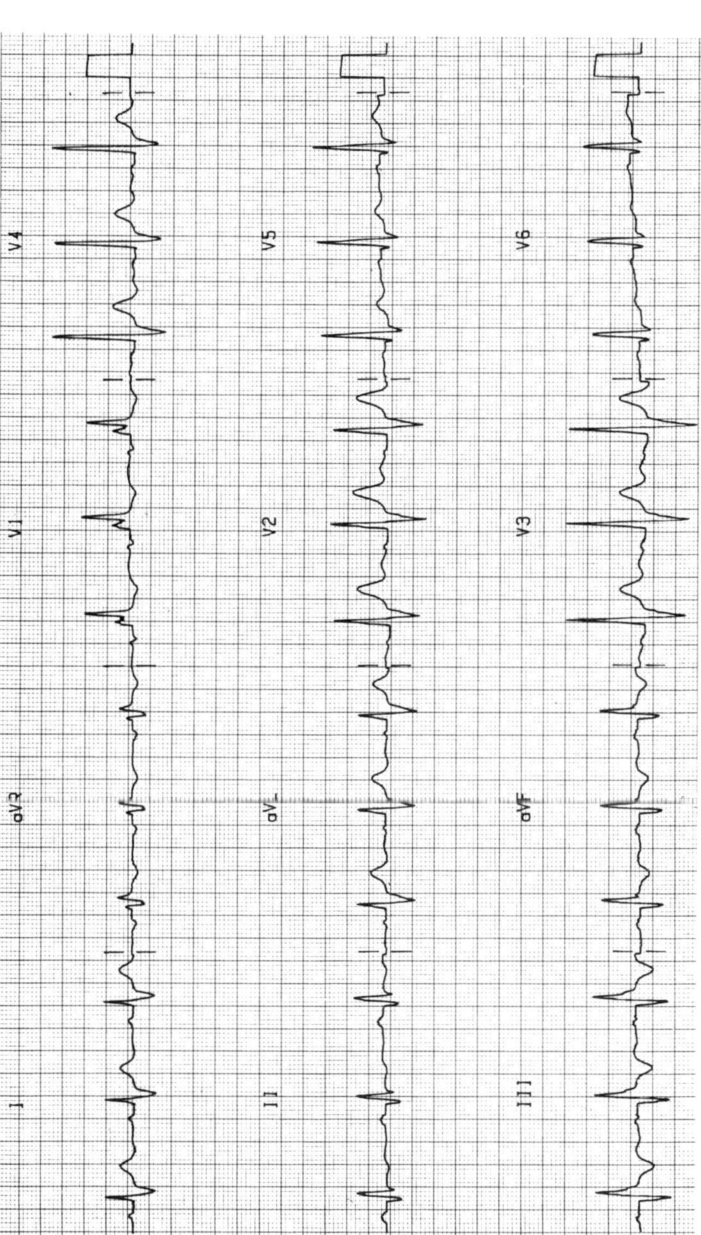

Figure 23: Right bundle branch block (RBBB). The QRS is broad (160 ms), with preceding P waves and a normal PR interval. The tall secondary R^1 wave in V1 and the S wave in V6 reflect late activation of the right ventricle. This patient also had sustained an inferior myocardial infarction (Q waves in II, III, and AV$_F$), illustrating that such a diagnosis is possible in the setting of RBBB.

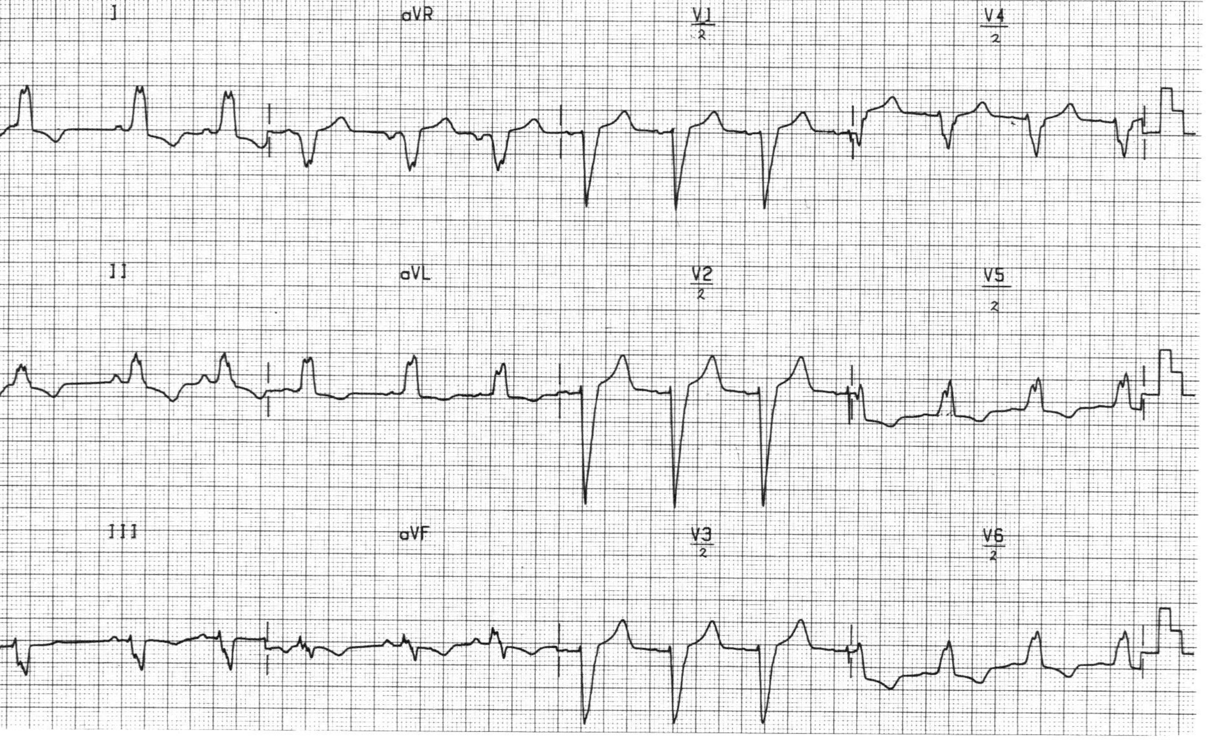

Figure 24: Left bundle branch block (LBBB). The QRS is broad (160 ms) and bizarre. The first beat recorded in AV_R, AV_L, and AV_F is an atrial ectopic beat, as diagnosed by the premature and abnormal preceding P wave.

pacing is almost always required. This grave situation is associated with a considerable mortality despite supportive measures.

Bundle branch blocks

The bundle branch blocks are quite different from the AV conduction disturbances already discussed. They are thought to be generated by problems within the ramifications of either the right or left bundle branches, producing a characteristic ECG appearance. Both alter activation of the ventricular myocardium (Figures 23 and 24). Ventricular activation time is prolonged. This might be expected to have implications for hemodynamic performance, but in reality the effect is trivial.

Right or left bundle branch block is hardly ever noticed by an affected patient. Right bundle branch block occurs in approximately 1 in 1000 individuals as an apparently normal variation. Left bundle branch block has never been considered a normal variant, but there may be isolated instances in which it is consistent with normal cardiac performance and a normal prognosis. The importance of the bundle branch blocks is their indication of potentially serious underlying heart disease. They are of particular significance if their manifestation is progressive.

There is no specific treatment for the bundle branch blocks, but their electrocardiographic pattern is important and should be recognized.

References

1. Bjerregaard P. The quality of ambulatory ECG-recordings and accuracy of semi-automatic arrhythmia analysis: An evaluation of the Medilog-Pathfinder system. Eur Heart J 1980;1:417-425.
2. The Cardiac Arrhythmia Suppression Trial Investigators. Preliminary report: effect of encainide and flecainide on mortality in a randomized trial of arrhythmia suppression after myocardial infarction. N Engl J Med 1989;321:406-412.
3. Bruce RA, De Rouen T, Peterson DR, et al. Noninvasive predictors of sudden cardiac death in men with coronary heart disease: predictive value of maximal stress testing. Am J Cardiol 1977;39:833-840.
4. Krahn AD, Manfreda J, Tate RB, et al. The natural-history of atrial-fibrillation: incidence, risk-factors, and prognosis in the Manitoba follow-up study. Am J Med 1995;98:476-484.
5. Anonymous. Warfarin versus aspirin for prevention of thromboembolism in atrial fibrillation: Stroke Prevention in Atrial Fibrillation II Study. Lancet 1994; 343:687-691.
6. Coumel P, Leclercq JF, Attuel P, et al. Autonomic influences in the genesis of atrial arrhythmias: atrial flutter and fibrillation of vagal origin. In: Narula OS, ed. Cardiac arrhythmias: electrophysiology, diagnosis and management. Baltimore: Williams and Wilkins, 1971:200-251.
7. Campbell RWF. Atrial fibrillation: steering a management course between thromboembolism and proarrhythmic risk. Eur Heart J 1995;16(suppl G):28-31.

8. Feld GK. Radiofrequency catheter ablation versus modification of the AV node for control of rapid ventricular response in atrial fibrillation. J Cardiovasc Electrophysiol 1995;6:217-228.

9. Halinen MO, Huttunen M, Paakkinen S, Tarssanen L. Comparison of sotalol with digoxin-quinidine for conversion of acute atrial fibrillation to sinus rhythm (the Sotalol-Digoxin-Quinidine Trial). Am J Cardiol 1995;76(7):495-498.

10. Reimold SC, Cantillon CO, Friedman PL, Antman EM. Propafenone versus sotalol for suppression of recurrent symptomatic atrial fibrillation. Am J Cardiol 1993;71(7):558-563.

11. Madrid AH, Moro C, Marin-Huerta E, et al. Comparison of flecainide and procainamide in cardioversion of atrial fibrillation. Eur Heart J 1993;14(8): 1127-1131.

12. Horner SM. A comparison of cardioversion of atrial fibrillation using oral amiodarone, intravenous amiodarone and DC cardioversion. Acta Cardiologica 1992;47(5):473-480.

13. Di Bianco R, Morganroth J, Freitag RJ, et al. Effects of Nadalol on the spontaneous and exercise provoked heart rate in patients with chronic atrial fibrillation receiving stable doses of digoxin. Am Heart J 1984;108:1121-1127.

14. Roth A, Harrison E, Mitani G, et al. Efficacy and safety of medium and high dose diltiazem alone and in combination with digoxin for control of heart rate at rest and during exercise in patients with chronic atrial fibrillation. Circulation 1986;73:316-324.

15. Feld GK, Fleck RP, Fujimura O, et al. Control of rapid ventricular response by radiofrequency catheter modification of the atrioventricular node in patients with medically refractory atrial fibrillation. Circulation 1994;90(5):2299-2307.

16. Cox JL, Boineau JP, Schuessler RB, et al. Modification of the Maze procedure for atrial flutter and atrial fibrillation. I. Rationale and surgical results. J Thorac Cardiovasc Surg 1995;110(2):473-484.

17. Waldo AL. Atrial flutter. New directions in management and mechanism. Circulation 1990;81(3):1142-1143.

18. Kirkorian G, Moncada E, Chevalier P, et al. Radiofrequency ablation of atrial flutter: efficacy of an anatomically guided approach. Circulation 1994;90(6): 2804-2814.

19. Muller G, Deal BJ, Benson DW. "Vagal maneuvers" and adenosine for termination of atrioventricular reentrant tachycardia. Am J Cardiol 1994;74:500-503.

20. Jackman WM, Wang XZ, Friday KJ, et al. Catheter ablation of accessory atrioventricular pathways (Wolff-Parkinson-White syndrome) by radiofrequency current. N Engl J Med 1991;324(23):1605-1611.

21. Klein GJ, Bashore TM, Sellers TD, et al. Ventricular fibrillation in the Wolff-Parkinson-White syndrome. N Engl J Med 1979;301:1080-1085.

22. McGuire MA, Ross DL, Uther JB, et al. Surgical procedure for the cure of atrioventricular junctional ("AV node") reentrant tachycardia: anatomic and electrophysiologic effects of dissection of the anterior atrionodal connections in a canine model. J Am Coll Cardiol 1994;24:784-794.
23. Kay GN, Epstein AE, Dailey SM, Plumb VJ. Selective radiofrequency ablation of the slow pathway for the treatment of atrioventricular nodal reentrant tachycardia: evidence for involvement of perinodal myocardium within the reentrant circuit. Circulation 1992;85(5):1675-1688.
24. Lesh MD, Van Hare GF, Epstein LM, et al. Radiofrequency catheter ablation of atrial arrhythmias: results and mechanisms. Circulation 1994;89(3):1074-1089.
25. Lown B, Fakhro AM, Hood WB, Thorn GW. The coronary care unit: new perspectives and directions. JAMA 1967;19:188-198.
26. Campbell RWF, Murray A, Julian DG. Ventricular arrhythmias in the first 12 hours of acute myocardial infarction: natural history study. Br Heart J 1981; 46:351-357.
27. Bigger JT, Fleiss JL, Kleiger R, et al. The relationships among ventricular arrhythmias, left ventricular dysfunction, and mortality in the two years after myocardial infarction. Circulation 1984;69:250-258.
28. Chizner MA, Pearle DL, de Leon AC. The natural history of aortic stenosis in adults. Am Heart J 1980;99:419-424.
29. Rae AP, Speilman SR, Kutalek SP, et al. Electrophysiologic assessment of antiarrhythmic drug efficacy for ventricular tachyarrhythmias associated with dilated cardiomyopathy. Am J Cardiol 1987;59:291-295.
30. The Cardiac Arrhythmia Suppression Trial II Investigators. Effect of the antiarrhythmic agent moricizine on survival after myocardial infarction. N Engl J Med 1992;327:227-233.
31. IMPACT Research Group. International mexiletine and placebo antiarrhythmic coronary trial: 1. Report on arrhythmia and other findings. J Am Coll Cardiol 1984;4(6):1148-1163.
32. Waldo AL, Camm AJ, deRuyter H, al et. for the SWORD investigators. Effect of d-sotalol on mortality in patients with left ventricular dysfunction after recent and remote myocardial infarction. Lancet 1996;348:7-12.
33. Cullen K, Stenhouse NS, Wearne KL, Cumpston GN. Electrocardiograms and 13 year cardiovascular mortality in Busselton study. Br Heart J 1982;47:209-210.
34. Levi GF, Proto C. Ventricular fibrillation in the course of Prinzmetal's angina pectoris: report of two cases. Br Heart J 1973;35(6):601-603.
35. Sarter BH, Finkle JK, Gerszten RT, Buxton AE. What is the risk of sudden cardiac death in patients presenting with hemodynamically stable sustained

ventricular tachycardia after myocardial infarction? J Am Coll Cardiol 1996;28: 122-129.

36. Anderson JL. Contemporary clinical trials in ventricular tachycardia and fibrillation: implications of ESVEM, CASCADE and CASK for clinical management. J Cardiovasc Electrophysiol 1995;6:880-886.

37. Waller TJ, Kay HR, Spielman SR, et al. Reduction in sudden death and total mortality by antiarrhythmic therapy evaluated by electrophysiologic drug testing: criteria of efficacy in patients with sustained ventricular tachyarrhythmia. J Am Coll Cardiol 1987;10(1):83-89.

38. Bourke JP, Campbell RWF, Renzulli A. Surgery for ventricular tachyarrhythmias based on fragmentation mapping in sinus rhythm alone. Eur J Cardiothorac Surg 1989;3:401-407.

39. Ector H, Jordaens L, Vanhaecke J. Survival analysis and clinical medicine: an observational comparison of the implantable cardioverter-defibrillator, amiodarone treatment and heart-transplantation. Eur Heart J 1996;17(9):1444-1447.

40. Gonska BD, Cao K, Schaumann A, et al. Catheter ablation of ventricular tachycardia in 136 patients with coronary artery disease: results and long-term follow-up. J Am Coll Cardiol 1994;24(6):1506-1514.

41. Rossi P, Massumi A, Gillette P, Hall RJ. Arrhythmogenic right ventricular dysplasia: clinical features, diagnostic techniques and current management. Am Heart J 1982;103:415-420.

42. Jadonath RL, Schwatzman DS, Preminger MV, et al. Utility of the 12 lead electrocardiogram in localizing the origin of right ventricular outflow tract tachycardia. Am Heart J 1995;130:1107-1113.

43. Klein LS, Shih H-T, Hackett K, et al. Radiofrequency catheter ablation of ventricular tachycardia in patients without structural heart disease. Circulation 1992;85:1666-1674.

44. McKenna WJ, Harris L, Perez G, et al. Arrhythmias in hypertrophic cardiomyopathy. II. Comparison of amiodarone and verapamil in treatment. Br Heart J 1981;46:173-178.

45. Dessertenne F. La tachycardia ventriculaire à deux foyers opposés variables. Arc Mal Coeur 1966;59:263.

46. Jervell A, Lange-Neilson F. Congenital deaf mutism, functional heart disease with prolongation of the QT interval, and sudden death. Am Heart J 1957; 54:59-68.

47. Kerem B, Benhorin J, Kalman YM, et al. Evidence for genetic heterogeneity in the long QT syndrome. Am J Hum Genet 1992;51:A192.

48. Moss AJ, Schwartz PJ, Crampton RS, et al. The long QT syndrome: prospective longitudinal study of 328 families. Circulation 1991;84:1136-1144.

49. Tzivoni D, Keren A, Cohen AM, et al. Magnesium therapy for torsade de pointes. Am J Cardiol 1984;53:528-30.

50. Sanna G, Arcidicacono R. Chemical ventricular defibrillation of the human heart with bretylium tosylate. Am J Cardiol 1973;32:982-987.

51. Koster RW, Dunning AJ. Intramuscular lidocaine for prevention of lethal arrhythmias in the prehospitalization phase of acute myocardial infarction. N Engl J Med 1985;313:1105-1110.

52. Emergency Cardiac Care Committee and Sub-Committees, American Heart Association. Guidelines for cardiopulmonary resuscitation and emergency cardiac care. J Am Med Assoc 192;268:2171-2302.

53. Shaw DB, Kekwick CA, Veake D, et al. Survival in second degree atrioventricular block. Br Heart J 1985;53:587-593.